Hepatitis C
SURVIVAL SECRETS

Medical accolades for this book:

"I believe *Hepatitis C Survival Secrets* and its accompanying website will dramatically help you and others with Hepatitis C to make the best and most informed choices regarding your treatment and your health. Be sure to consider all it contains very carefully. This book gets my highest recommendation."
– *Vikki Shaw, Ph.D.*

"A thoughtful, intelligent and comprehensive guide to navigating the therapeutic options for overcoming chronic Hepatitis C infection."
– *Leo Galland, M.D.,*
   Director, Foundation for Integrated Medicine

"I have known Ralph Napolitano for over eight years as he has researched ways to protect and support his liver from the ravages of Hepatitis C. During his quest, Ralph has helped thousands of others deal with this potentially deadly condition. This book, *Hepatitis C Survival Secrets*, is his latest contribution to helping others with Hepatitis C. I highly recommend it."
– *Dan Wen, M.D. (China)*

"Ralph Napolitano has done a unique and exemplary service in writing *Hepatitis C Survival Secrets*. He has assembled substantial evidence regarding the best approaches for dealing with this disease. If you or a loved one has Hepatitis C, you simply must read this book."
– *Dean Shrock, Ph.D., author of*
   Why Love Heals and Doctor's Orders: Go Fishing

"One of the greatest tragedies in our current healthcare system is the ever-increasing number of Americans who want (but are not receiving) intelligent discussion, straightforward presentations of options and, most of all, a sense that someone really cares in relation to their health concerns. In *Hepatitis C Survival Secrets*, Ralph Napolitano provides all this and more for the many in our society suffering from Hepatitis C."
– *Dr. Jeffrey Moss, co-author of*
   Textbook of Nutritional Medicine

Hepatitis C
SURVIVAL SECRETS

WITH CRITICAL INSIGHTS
YOUR DOCTOR WON'T SHARE

Ralph Napolitano
Hepatitis C Survivor,
Licensed Health Care Practitioner
and Health Researcher

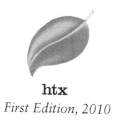

htx
First Edition, 2010

HEPATITIS C SURVIVAL SECRETS
With Critical Insights Your Doctor Won't Share

Editor: Rachel Danks, PhD., Medical Writing Consultancy

Design, Layout & Typography by Blair Saldanah
blair@saldanah.com

Body text typeset in Sabon, 10.5 on 15 – headings set in Clarendon.
Book built entirely on Apple computers with Adobe software and type.

ISBN 978-0-615-16628-5

Library of Congress Control Number: 2007938628

HTX Enterprises
PO Box 1549
Pine Bush, NY 12566
www.HepCSurvival.com

Dedication

To my family, both close and extended.
You know who you are. Please know that I love you.

Also, to you, the reader and the millions of
others "surviving" Hepatitis C today.

Most of all I want to acknowledge
my Mom and Dad, for giving me life, and my children,
Lia and Michael, for making it worth living.

Disclaimer

This book contains the opinions and ideas of the author
(along with input from other Hepatitis C survivors).

The contents are intended to provide helpful and instructive
information on the subject of Hepatitis C.

This book is sold with the understanding that the author is
not engaged in rendering medical, health, or any other kind of
personal professional services in the book.

The reader should consult with his or her medical or
healthcare professional before adopting any of the suggestions
in this book, or drawing their own conclusions from it.

The author specifically disclaims all responsibility for any liability,
loss or risk, personal or otherwise, which might be incurred
as a consequence, directly or indirectly, of the use and application
of any of the contents of this book.

Acknowledgements

Dr. Edward Croen, my gastroenterologist, for respecting my opinions about my personal health and how best to deal with it, while at the same time providing me with the best medical advice and care possible.

Dr. Leo Galland, for graciously answering my questions about Hepatitis C and Complementary and Alternative medicine for well over 12 years now.

Dr. Jeffrey Moss, who continues to inspire me with his dedication to learning more and sharing more about improving health through nutritional supplementation.

Vikki Shaw, Ph.D., for working tirelessly to provide a valuable resource for all "survivors."

Alan Franciscus, publisher and of the *HCV Advocate,* a national HCV patient newsletter and the web site: *www.hcvadvocate.org,* for giving me invaluable input when needed early on.

Kevin and Patty Krueger, of The National Hepatitis C Coalition, *www.nationalhepatitis-c.org* for thirteen years of helping me and so many other patients, in so many ways.

Dr. Stephen Levine, for input over the years that has been more valuable than he could even imagine.

Ms. Megan Rooney, for unflagging assistance in answering my toughest nutritional supplement questions over the years.

Mr. William Meyer, for helping me get started with production of the world's best Milk Thistle product in 1999 and helping make the more powerful **MegaThistle** even more affordable in 2010.

Mr. Bob Korngold, creative guide and much more. Thanks for sharing your big heart and brilliant mind.

Mr. Paul Puskas, for his knowledgeable advice about the good, the bad and the dangerous in the nutritional supplement industry.

Mr. Chet Holmes, for being an incredible inspiration, mentor, and friend, for over twenty-seven years.

Joanna Cook Napolitano, for being a great mother to our children, and for her encouragement, support and initiative in helping me help so many people with Hepatitis C.

CONTENTS

Foreword by
Vikki Shaw, Ph.D.

Welcome to "Hepatitis C Survival Secrets". In my humble opinion you have in your hands one of the best books ever written for Hepatitis C survivors (like you and me).

My name is Vikki Shaw, and our paths may have crossed on the internet over the years. That's where I met Ralph Napolitano, the author of this book, about ten years ago.

Allow me to give you some background. In 1998 I individually started and personally ran the largest and most popular private website for helping people learn about Hepatitis C. I feverishly built the site to over 2,500 pages in just a few short years. It was a labor of love. This was totally non-commercial.

As a Hepatitis C survivor and avid researcher (like Ralph) I wanted to help others come to grips with this disease as best I could. I knew there wasn't enough good, reliable information out there. Even today, nearly forty government and education sites link to my original website, for the valuable information it contains.

From the beginning, my site was populated with articles from medical journals and other sources people would not normally have access to (along with my own commentary and recommended resources). The subscriptions to the medical journals alone cost me a small fortune, but I was dedicated to helping others, so I absorbed the cost.

As part of the site I also started a support forum, and I strongly recommend that you become involved in one yourself, if you are not already. Ralph intends to have a forum available as part of the "Hepatitis C Survival Secrets" website *http://www.HepCSurvival. com* (more on that later). Be sure to sign in there and connect with other survivors. If you are like most people, you will find the support invaluable to your well-being.

Even though I have not been directly involved with my original website for years now (I'll explain later), I still have a very strong reason to want to help you sort out the good stuff from the bull.

You see, six years previous to starting my website I was told by my doctors that I had end-stage liver disease due to chronic Hepatitis C, and that I should put my affairs in order because I was fast approaching a rapid decline leading to my imminent death. Well, clearly, the prognosis of my impending death was greatly exaggerated (after all, that was over 15 years ago). As of this writing I am still alive and kicking, and some would say, just as cantankerous as ever. That's part of the reason I've always liked Ralph's attitude that those of us still alive with Hepatitis C are "survivors".

My experience with my physicians, though, showed me how little the doctors themselves knew. While doctors may know a bit more now, what they know and how much they share with patients is still questionable to me. That's why I still feel it is imperative to further educate and inform others who also have this potentially deadly disease, as Ralph has so capably done with this book.

As part of my internet mission to inform and enlighten others, who, like myself, were dealing with Hepatitis C, I sent out regular email alerts to visitors of my site who chose to subscribe to my updates (and I also posted to my forum regularly, fielding questions and providing whatever support I could).

It was in 1999 that I was contacted by Ralph, as one of my subscribers. He told me how valuable he thought my work was on behalf of the Hepatitis C community and how appreciative he was for what I was doing. (I was actually accustomed to hearing that quite a bit from website visitors and update subscribers.)

During our conversation Ralph asked me what I thought about milk thistle for people with liver concerns. I told him that I believed it could have considerable value, based on the research I had seen, but that my body could not tolerate the herb for some reason. I had tried it on more than one occasion and ingesting it actually made me feel ill.

It was then that he mentioned this new form of milk thistle he was making available online to Hepatitis C patients through a business he and his wife, Joanna, had started. He explained this product isolated the most powerful liver protective constituent of milk thistle and bound it to a substance that increased absorption by up to 1,000 percent (on its own, milk thistle is notoriously hard to absorb – for instance, milk thistle tea is essentially worthless for anyone with real liver concerns).

Ralph went on to explain the product he was introducing was much more like a medicine than an herb and sent me the clinical study results which fully supported that position (my Ph.D. is in the medical field, so I know how to interpret clinical studies). He wondered if I'd like to give his new product a try to see if it might not have a negative effect on me that other milk thistle products did. I agreed to test it out. Obviously, I already trusted this guy seeing as I had just agreed to be a research guinea pig for him.

Much to my surprise, not only did this product NOT make me feel ill, I actually felt a marked improvement in just a couple of weeks. Given the results I experienced first-hand, I was convinced Ralph had found something of great value for protecting and supporting the liver without any negative side effects. I began recommending the product to my email list and many, many people thanked me for the positive impact it had on their health.

Over the ensuing years, Ralph and I became internet and telephone buddies. He and I were both in constant contact with other Hep C survivors, and continued helping them as best we could. When my life started to move in another direction and I realized I could no longer maintain my website, Ralph and Joanna stepped up to take over and keep it running for me.

Over the time I had already known him, Ralph had proven to me that he is a man of integrity who really cares about helping others with Hepatitis C to the best of his ability. As a licensed healthcare provider, helping people is one of his primary objectives in life. In my opinion, this book is further proof of the depth of his caring concern. He recognizes there is still a need to help people most easily determine the best course of action for themselves regarding this disease.

Ralph is an intelligent and inquisitive individual. Through ongoing research and investigation, he went on to discover which other natural means would be of most value to people with Hepatitis C. He then did his best to make any appropriate products he discovered available at the lowest possible cost. And, at the same time he kept looking for additional valuable information regarding lifestyle, nutrition, etc., and providing the results of his ardent research to other people at no cost. Like me, he personally communicated with thousands of other Hepatitis C survivors through his websites, email and even over the telephone.

Also, like me, Ralph has chosen not to go the medical route of treatment because he has genotype 1 (the toughest type of HCV to treat with current medical therapy, and also the most common in North America, representing about 70 to 80 percent of those infected). He never directly dissuades people from choosing such therapy, he just informs them of other things they could do to protect and support their ailing livers most effectively and efficiently (regardless of whatever other choice they may make regarding treatment). Incidentally, Ralph's "A-List" of nutritional supplement recommendations is probably the best you can find anywhere, to protect and support you and your liver most efficiently and cost-effectively.

Three-and-a-half years ago Ralph and Joanna divorced and he left their company, signing a multi-year agreement stating he would not be involved in the Hepatitis C realm. This was a very tough time in his life. As much as helping others with Hepatitis C was important to him, he was constrained from continuing to do so.

However, that agreement has expired and Joanna recently sold the enterprise to a couple of "businessmen". Now, Ralph is back doing what he feels very strongly about, helping other people like you and I to deal with Hepatitis C in the best ways possible (and offering the most powerful liver-support supplements at the lowest possible price – something his former company seems to have lost sight of).

I believe "Hepatitis C Survival Secrets" and its accompanying website will dramatically help you and others with Hepatitis C to make the best and most informed choices regarding your treatment and your health. Be sure to consider all it contains very carefully. This book gets my highest recommendation.

As I always say, "Idle time is Hepatitis C's best friend." So don't just sit there, do something. Reading "Hepatitis C Survival Secrets" and following the advice it contains can help to keep you busy in very positive ways. Then just keep moving forward.

My wish for you is that you continue to survive Hepatitis C, enjoy your life, and leave this earth peacefully from natural causes at a very old age.

– *Vikki Shaw, Ph.D.*
January, 2010

As its title infers, this book truly includes Hepatitis C survival "secrets". And, though many of these secrets are hidden in plain sight in various places, some are not at all well known, and many are never shared by doctors with their patients. These secrets most certainly need to be in the awareness of all Hepatitis C survivors.

This book brings these secrets together in one place.

With its focus on survival secrets, this book also contains an overall message of hope.

Actual survivor stories are dispersed throughout this book. To read more survivor stories, (or to add your own stories or secrets) go to *http://www.HepCSurvival.com/stories.*

Your involvement there could be of genuine help to both yourself *and* others. – *Ralph*

Survival Secrets
Introduction

The odds of surviving this
disease are already high,
and YOU can increase them.

Assuming that you're reading this book because you or a loved one has chronic Hepatitis C, the fact that the virus doesn't really want to kill you should offer some cause for optimism. Biologically, viruses actually want to keep the host alive so they can continue to replicate. If a "smart" virus wants to keep you alive, I hope mine is a "genius". The chronic part of Hepatitis C just means you've had the infection in your body more than six months.

DEFINITION OF A HEPATITIS C SURVIVOR

As trite as this may sound, anyone living with Hepatitis C is a survivor – no matter how they are dealing with the illness. If you're alive today, you ARE surviving thus far. As frightening and potentially life-threatening as the disease can be, statistics show that you're more likely to die of old age than from liver failure or other problems associated with Hepatitis C. Because the liver is a non-complaining organ, many patients live normal, asymptomatic (symptom-less) lives for 10, 20 or 30 years before they even learn they have the disease! For this reason Hepatitis C is often called a "silent epidemic". In fact, it is estimated that only half the people who are infected in North America know they are.

GENERAL HEPATITIS C VIRUS INFORMATION

There are an estimated 200 million people worldwide (yes, two hundred million) infected with the Hepatitis C virus (HCV). That's *3.3 percent* of the world's population. This prevalence makes it one of the greatest worldwide threats to public health ever faced.

Up to five million people in the U.S. are infected with Hepatitis C. Sixty-five percent of those infected are between 30 and 49 years of age.

The U.S. National Institutes for Health estimate four million Americans have the infection, but most researchers say that number is closer to five million.

In the U.S.A., Hepatitis C is *five-times more prevalent* than AIDS and around ten thousand Americans die annually as a result of HCV infection (and that number is expected to *triple* by 2019). Chronic liver disease is the tenth leading cause of death in the U.S. and studies indicate 40 to 60 percent of these are related to HCV.

> Again, the most important secret about Hepatitis C is that it's NOT fatal to the vast majority of sufferers.

Survivor Story:

"Along the way I see that some people have NO idea that they can put off treatment if their liver isn't in too bad shape and they aren't suffering. A lot of people think they have no choice but to treat. I try to tell them otherwise, to do their research and make their decision from there. Many people go into treatment immediately after diagnosis, like after their very first visit to the doctor, which I find appalling. I feel their doctors don't give them much choice."

– Barry

Survivor Story:

"I am very lucky, though I do get depressed because I have Hep C. I say I am lucky because I have had it for about 35 years without symptoms. I did not respond to Pegasys & Rebetrol unfortunately. I am between stage 2 and 3 and have genotype 4. My viral load and enzyme levels are very low and doc says I will die with this and not from it. The latest statistics are now out, and after 30 years post-infection 75 percent do not even have cirrhosis. Most people do OK with this and I guess I am one of the lucky ones. I guess I should thank God every day but I still get angry and depressed and frightened that I even have it. I wish they could cure me, but yet I have to be grateful because I am one of the lucky ones. Most people ought to focus on the statistics. That way they may not get so bent out of shape."
– Kitty

BASIC LIVER FACTS

Your liver is your largest internal organ (skin being your largest organ overall). Your liver is located on the right side of your lower rib cage. About the size of a football, it takes care of approximately 500 vital bodily functions. It processes practically everything you take into your body.

Along with converting food to energy, creating building blocks for cells, hormones and immune factors, among many other functions, the liver also stores some nutrients for later use, and detoxifies any harmful substances. It is also regenerative; three-quarters of a healthy liver can be removed and will grow back within weeks.

HEPATITIS C VIRUS SURVIVAL FACTS

According to the Centers for Disease Control and Prevention, only 20 to 30 percent of Chronic Hepatitis C patients will develop life-threatening complications, meaning 70 to 80 percent will lead relatively normal lives.

These encouraging statistics don't mean you shouldn't take responsibility for your health and happiness. You can and you should. That's why I've written this book – to provide an overview of some of the best approaches available. These include conventional "Western" medicine, natural and herbal remedies, Chinese, Japanese and Ayurvedic medicine, as well as dietary supplements, stress-reduction techniques and more. In addition, I'd like to help you avoid the assorted quacks and "snake-oil" salesmen who promise cures for a disease that (as of today) has NO proven natural cure.

HOW DID I COME BY MY "KNOWLEDGE"?

Well, along with being a veteran healthcare provider, licensed in New York since 1981, I'm also a Hepatitis C survivor. Additionally, I've communicated directly with well over a thousand other Hepatitis C patients through the websites I started and ran to be of service to the Hepatitis C community, beginning in 1999. Although I am no longer involved with these websites, I directly and indirectly helped many thousands of Hepatitis C survivors over the years.

The original concept for this book was simply as a collection of survivor stories. I sent an email to thousands of patients and got back hundreds of replies. It was in reading these stories and speaking to other survivors that I realized there was still so much disinformation and misinformation out there. There were facts that should be common knowledge but still seemed to be escaping many patients' awareness. This is when the element of sharing these survival "secrets" entered the picture.

Also, just to bind up hundreds of stories and offer them as a book didn't seem to be as good as an idea once I had the stories in hand. There was quite a lot of repetition and many were poorly written. So, I decided to use just the most relevant, instead.

Some of the full text stories are still available to you, though, at the website *http://www.HepCSurvival.com/stories* As stated earlier, if you want to read more stories, that is the place to go (you'll also be able to share your own personal story or comment on the stories that appear there already).

My Story (the abbreviated version)

Like many patients, I discovered my illness by accident. In 1989, I applied for an increase to my life insurance plan. Needless to say, I was shocked when my insurance agent told me I'd been denied extra coverage because of my blood test. He didn't have any specifics, but tried to reassure me by saying, "Don't worry, Ralph, we all have to go sometime." Clearly, this was less than reassuring.

Later, when I discovered the problem was elevated liver enzymes, I was determined to find out why. Unfortunately, my chosen doctor (recommended by my insurance agent) was "in over his head." At our first meeting, he kept asking if I was experiencing night sweats. Finally, after the fourth time he asked, I inquired why he wanted to know. He told me that night sweats were a possible sign of non-Hodgkin's lymphoma. He assumed I had CANCER.

After much fumbling and bumbling, follow-up appointments and tests, I was diagnosed with non-A, non-B Hepatitis (this was before the Hepatitis C Virus was isolated).

Now, the only time in my life I'd had active Hepatitis was at age 20, several weeks after giving blood. The blood drive was conducted in the basement of our county center, and I guess they were careless about sterilizing equipment. If you're interested, you can read more about my story at *http://www.HepCSurvival.com*.

SURVIVAL SECRET

Do your research; learn as much as you can. Having more information will further empower you.

More Information Gives You More Options

Some of the best advice I can give you is to become as educated as possible about Hepatitis C. You must take responsibility for your decisions regarding this disease, and that starts with being as informed as possible. From the moment I learned about my elevated liver enzymes, I began treating myself holistically. I researched all the literature I could find regarding liver disease, conventional treatment and natural healing. I combed the library, and once it became available, I dived into the internet. I consulted with naturopaths, homeopaths, clinical nutritionists, and holistic MDs, amongst others. I even had a local cable television show where I interviewed many of these experts.

One of the first nutritional supplement products I chose was milk thistle extract, because so much had been written about its centuries-long success with liver ailments. There is no other herb that has such an impressive reputation for liver support and protection. While I knew from my research that milk thistle alone would not directly treat or cure the disease or fight the virus in any way, I wanted to protect and support my liver as best I could through natural means. I'll discuss milk thistle – especially its most effective type, the phytosome form of milk thistle found in MegaThistle – along with other effective natural products in Chapter 3. For now, suffice it so say that the phytosome form of milk thistle remains at the center of my treatment universe, despite the fact that I've refined and augmented my regimen over the decades. I feel very strongly that everyone who suffers from Hepatitis C should have access to this powerful supplement, which is why I have developed and highly recommend the new, powerful and much more affordable brand of the phytosome form. As stated above, this new product is called MegaThistle.

IMPORTANT PERSONAL NOTE

Although I touch on my own wellness regimen throughout the book, I will not prescribe a specific course of treatment for anyone. Even if I ignored individual differences in factors such as immune response, overall health, diet, and family history, the Hepatitis C virus has six major genetic strains (genotypes) and at least 15 different subtypes. In my opinion, this discredits the notion of a one-size-fits-all approach – at least for now. Current research with protease inhibitors and other biochemical substances may soon,

I hope, change that opinion. And, other viable treatment approaches may be just over the horizon. However, in my opinion, the current medical therapy (Interferon plus Ribavirin) is best avoided by those, like myself, with genotype 1. Its sucess rate is just too low.

Survivor Story:

"I feel fortunate not only because my AST/ALT levels remain far within the "normal" range but also because my genotype, 2b, is said to achieve higher success rate with current treatment, although that does not interest me at this time. I am waiting on a treatment that is less caustic, if it ever becomes available. I know someone who has gone through treatment and I cannot afford a cure that is worse than the illness (yet)."
    – Verde

Survivor Story:

"I am waiting for a better treatment to become available, with better results than the current treatment, which is very low in effectiveness and very high in side effects – especially with my genotype, 1a. I hope research will now take a serious look at this epidemic as it has for HIV, and fund appropriately."
    – Shelby

GENERAL TREATMENT OPTIONS

This book is based on decades of reading and research, including literally thousands of communications with other Hepatitis C survivors. Ultimately, my goal is to present the various treatment options that boast clinical, empirical and/or strong anecdotal evidence for supporting and improving liver function – at a reasonable cost. As stated throughout this book, I am not a big fan of the current medical therapy of Interferon plus Ribavirin, especially for those of us with genotype 1. (And, thankfully, neither are my doctors.)

SURVIVAL SECRET
You have choices.

Although I personally subscribe to natural remedies and lifestyle choices, I recognize that there is a place for conventional medical intervention, especially for patients whose illnesses are in the advanced stages, or who have certain genotypes. Current therapy is much more effective for genotype 2 or 3 than for other genotypes.

Unfortunately, experience has taught me that many patients are polarized along the following lines:

- Those who blindly follow "doctors' orders," without asking any questions or investigating alternative therapies; or

- Those who subscribe to an "anti-medical/pharmaceutical, conspiracy-theory approach," and promote just about anything that doesn't "jibe" with the conventional wisdom.

DOCTORS GENERALLY MEAN WELL, BUT...

On the one hand, I'd like to stress that, generally, doctors truly want to help you to the best of their ability. When you visit a doctor, she really wants to help you. (She may have only 10 minutes to help on any given day, but she genuinely wants to help.) For better or worse, however, your doctor is ethically and legally obliged to follow certain rules and guidelines with regard to treating your condition.

At the time of this writing, there is just one conventionally/ medically-approved treatment predominantly prescribed for chronic Hepatitis C – regardless of the virus's genotype and subtype, and no matter how far the disease has progressed. This treatment is Pegylated Interferon-Ribavirin combination therapy ("combo" therapy). The side effects range from mild, flu-like symptoms to the absolutely horrendous. Some people have experienced truly debilitating side effects. One woman sticks out in my mind – like me, she was asymptomatic (had no obvious symptoms of the disease) and her virus was genotype 1a. She didn't feel sick, but decided to start therapy on the advice of her doctor. She quickly developed nerve sensitivity, and was finally taken off the treatment early. This woman ended up in constant pain from acute peripheral neuropathy – to the point where, when I last spoke with her, she was dependent on opiates to relieve the pain, and was barely getting through life. This was a woman who'd been leading a very normal life until then. What happened to her wasn't necessary (nor usual). More currently (and more publicly), look at Natalie Cole, who experienced kidney failure and underwent a transplant *as a result of the medical treatment* for her Hepatitis C, not from the disease itself.

On the other hand, some people have experienced very beneficial results from this treatment – results approximating what most people would call a cure, although many people prefer to think of it as long-term remission.

Survivor Story:

"While hospitalized for an unrelated illness in 2003, a new doctor ran a Hep C test which came back positive. My viral load was 820,000 and I learned my genotype is 2. I also learned that there is treatment of which I only had vague knowledge up to that point. My first reaction was that I had heard the side effects were too bad. My very wise young doctor said "if it gets bad, you can stop".
So I stopped arguing and started treatment on March 20, 2004. I was treated with Pegasys and Copegasys. The side effects weren't too bad in the beginning and I made it through six months of treatment without missing a day of work. Today, so far, I am virus-free."
– Elizabeth

Survivor Story:

"I was put on Pegaysys injection once a week and Copegasys (five pills daily) for six months. I finished my six month treatment last week. I was virus free after month three. I was shocked all the way around. First, that I lasted on the drugs and second that the effects of the drugs did not kill me. I did experience the usual nausea, headache

and extreme fatigue, plus about ten other side effects
that are not too bad. Thank goodness the doctor gave me
medicine for the side effects. The different medications for
the side effects helped me out tremendously. I was able to
function most of the time and when I couldn't I would just
try to sleep and lay around."
     – Paul

SURVIVAL SECRET

As of this time, there is a website
developed by other Hepatitis C
survivors with information on
dealing with treatment side
effects from A to Z. It is:

www.hepcsurvivalguide.org.

While this site is perhaps a bit outdated, it is the best single source
of this particular type of information I have found. Incidentally,
I have no affiliation with the website, I simply approve of its
contents.

HOW THIS BOOK CAN HELP YOU

Even though I believe in natural remedies to protect and support
your liver, I recognize the possible benefits of conventional/medical
treatments. They work for some people (although often at the cost
of taking a real toll on the overall health of the individual during
treatment and beyond). I also recognize that some so-called "natural"
treatments are nothing but old-fashioned scams designed to relieve
"suckers" of their money. In addition, there are some remedies that
actually have value, created by some well-known practitioners, but
that are outrageously expensive.

Some practitioners of traditional Chinese medicine, for example, offer proprietary combinations of herbs that cost upwards of $1,200 per month – FOR HERBS! Granted, these are good herbs, and the physicians are dedicated "believers," but is it worth $1,200 per month? I think not. Especially when there is no way they are going to "cure" Hepatitis C with this approach.

For these reasons and more, every Hepatitis C survivor needs to learn about the myriad of strategies and approaches available to manage their illness. Some people choose to take the conventional medical approach simply because it's covered by health insurance; others choose alternative medications because they believe they will be better off: and still others bury their heads in the sand and do nothing.

By the way, doing nothing is always an option. However, I don't recommend it. The "ostrich approach" has no real benefit. Find a good healthcare provider experienced with Hepatitis C, and work closely with this person. And, get smart on the disease yourself (by reading this book and others, and by researching on the internet).

You can ignore the problem, you can run scared, or you can seek the best information available. Whatever you do, you qualify as a survivor as long as you stay alive. But isn't it better to become an educated and informed survivor, an active survivor – someone who takes control of his or her destiny – instead of just crossing your fingers?

To help you even more, I've included many stories from actual survivors throughout the book to make certain points easier for you to appreciate and/or understand (and to add a further human element to the reality of surviving Hepatitis C).

Here's to your ongoing health, healing, happiness, and hope,
Ralph Napolitano

CHAPTER 1

What Must You Know First?

Y

You probably already know the "basics" of Hepatitis C – e.g., the nature of the virus, its transmission, symptoms, progression, tests to determine liver enzyme levels and viral loads, etc. There are many other books out there that cover these basics for you. Therefore, you may be tempted to skip this chapter. Well, skip at your own risk. In the pages that follow, you may find some information and suggestions you've never encountered before. If you must, please "skim" until you reach the material you didn't know. Besides, it never hurts to review the basics.

And when I say *basics,* I mean *basics*. Because this is a practical guide to treatment options – not a biology or medical textbook – I focus only on what Hepatitis C patients need to know about the illness. If, for example, you'd like to learn more about how viruses reproduce, please consult the internet. Also, be sure to check out the Resources section of this book for more suggested research sources.

HEPATITIS B AND HEPATITIS A
VACCINATIONS

SURVIVAL SECRET

If you are diagnosed with Hepatitis C, get vaccinated for Hepatitis A and B immediately...

This is highly recommended if you don't already have the antibodies, which can be determined through blood testing.

A liver already sick with Hepatitis C can be devastated by concurrent viral infection with either Hepatitis A or B. Your doctor should routinely make this recommendation as soon as you are diagnosed with chronic Hepatitis C. If not, then the suggestion (demand) is yours to make. It could save your life.

HEPATITIS C VIRUS FACTS

Hepatitis simply means "liver inflammation"; from the Greek, "hepat" (liver) and "itis" (inflammation). The Hepatitis C virus (HCV), first isolated in 1998, is transmitted from person to person by direct contact with infected blood. Like some other types of hepatitis, Hepatitis C has two forms: acute and chronic.

Survivor Story:

"I am not, and have never been, an IV drug user, and never had any transfusions. The only way I can explain my illness is that when I joined the Marines, they used an air-jet gun on all of us in line for our inoculations."

– Ernie

Acute Hepatitis C occurs when the virus is first contracted and may last for several weeks. It may or may not have obvious symptoms. Symptoms of acute Hepatitis C usually occur within six to nine weeks after infection, and 15 to 25 percent of those infected rid their bodies of the virus within a year.

Unlike other Hepatitis viruses, however, HCV is more likely to cause the chronic (life-long) form of the disease. Of those infected, 75 to 85 percent develop chronic Hepatitis C.

Chronic Hepatitis C refers to the situation in which the body cannot eradicate the virus and the disease becomes an ongoing, long-term, and usually slowly progressing. (it officially becomes "chronic" at six months). About 20 to 30 percent of people with a chronic infection eventually develop cirrhosis (complete scarring of the liver), which puts them at high risk of liver failure or liver cancer. Fibrosis and cirrhosis are caused by damaged or destroyed liver cells being replaced with fibrotic tissue. The more the liver is scarred in this way, the less it is able to perform its many very important functions.

As fibrosis progresses to cirrhosis, complications may occur such as portal hypertension (high blood pressure in your key liver vein) or an accumulation of fluid in the abdomen, which is called ascites.

As damage proceeds further, one may experience esophageal varices (like varicose veins or hemorrhoids that occur in the throat) which can be life-threatening if they burst. One of the goals of this book is to help you minimize, or completely avoid, the risk of ever experiencing any such complications.

Prior to 1989, when donated blood was first screened for the virus, many people contracted Hepatitis C through blood transfusions. Once the tainted blood was removed from the U.S. blood supply, the rate of new infections began to decline dramatically. But, new infections are still occurring at an alarming rate.

Most experts believe Hepatitis C is now spreading through the following means of blood-to-blood transmission:

- Shared use of intravenous or "inhaled" drug paraphernalia.
- Tattoos or piercing.
- Mother-to-child transmission.
- Sharing items such as toothbrushes, nail files or razors with traces of contaminated blood.

- Occupational exposure, especially among physicians, nurses and other healthcare workers.
- Sexual transmission (very rare, and probably caused by high-risk sexual behavior involving blood-to-blood contact).

MORE ABOUT SEXUAL TRANSMISSION

Hepatitis C virus does not appear to be spread through semen or any sexual secretions, but rather through "rough sex" and any other sexual activities that involve blood-to-blood contact. The "high-risk" groups include participants in anal sex, men who have sex with men, people with many sex partners, sex workers, and people with sexually transmitted diseases.

According to the Centers for Disease Control, people in stable, long-term monogamous relationships do not need to change their sexual practices, provided they are not high-risk practices. The "high-risk" groups should take appropriate precautions, such as highly-durable condoms.

> *Survivor Story:*
> *"When I was first diagnosed with Type 1a, it is likely I had already had the disease for at least 10 years. That was about the time I got my tattoo. It was a shock, to say the least, since I had no symptoms."*
> *– Wendy*

SURVIVAL SECRET

If you are a U.S. Military Veteran, definitely get tested for HCV ASAP.

U.S. MILITARY VETERANS AND HCV

The incidence of chronic Hepatitis C infections in the U.S. is much greater among veterans, especially Vietnam-era veterans. One hypothesis to explain this is that the airgun inoculations commonly used at that time may not always have been sufficiently sterile to prevent the virus being passed on. There are other common risk factors among veterans, as well. *Veterans* magazine, from July/August 2009 stated that two-thirds of all HCV patients in the U.S. have served in the military.

According to the Department of Veterans Affairs, "One in ten U.S. veterans is infected with HCV". This 10 percent infection rate is more than five times higher than the general population, which is estimated at 1.8 percent.

If you are a veteran, it is strongly recommended that you get tested for HCV. Also, make that recommendation to all veterans you know. The Veterans Administration is there to help all veterans. For more detailed information, I suggest you visit *http://www.hcvets.com*.

COMMON SYMPTOMS

When first infected, people with acute Hepatitis C may experience flu-like symptoms (fever, aches and fatigue) or even jaundice, which causes the skin or eyes to become abnormally yellow. On the other hand, they may be asymptomatic (having no symptoms at all), or develop mild symptoms that are easily confused with those of another illness. If the disease becomes chronic, you may develop some – but probably not all – of the following symptoms[1]:

- Fatigue: this is the most commonly reported symptom.
- Digestive problems: nausea, vomiting, diarrhea, bloating, gas, indigestion, abdominal pain, loss of appetite.
- Emotional problems: depression, anxiety, mood swings.
- Flu-like symptoms: headache, low-grade fever, night sweats, chills, joint and muscle pain, weakness.
- Hormonal problems: more intense premenstrual tension or menopausal symptoms, irregular periods, loss of sex drive, erectile dysfunction.
- Jaundice: yellowing of the skin or eyes, dark urine, pale or clay-colored stools.
- Skin problems: dry skin, itchy skin, bruising, reddened palms, red spidery spots, swelling of the hands, feet or face.
- Insomnia.
- Cognitive (thinking) problems: brain fog, encephalopathy (severe brain/cognitive problems with cirrhosis.

1 From *Living with Hepatitis C for Dummies*, Nina L. Paul, Ph.D., Hoboken, NJ: Wiley Publishing, Inc., 2005.

Again, hepatitis simply describes a swelling of the liver. Ironically, it's your body's own immune system that causes this swelling. In an effort to kill the invading viruses, your system's antibodies also damage cells in the liver – the biochemical reactions that accompany this process can also cause swelling. If this process continues for a long period, fibrosis (scarring) will occur, followed by extensive scarring, or cirrhosis.

Symptoms of cirrhosis can include: ascites (mentioned earlier); swelling of the legs; small red blood vessels visible on the surface of the skin; bleeding hemorrhoids; decreased urination; nosebleed or bleeding gums; breast development in men; bone loss and/or severe itching caused by the build-up of toxins (and high bilirubin levels).[2]

SURVIVAL SECRET

For those newly infected – some research suggests the best time to get treated is within the shortest time possible from the time of initial infection.

Newly-Infected?

If you can be treated within the initial active phase of the disease, your odds of obtaining a "cure" (sustained virological response) are improved. This makes sense because treatment can boost your body's initial immune response, creating a greater possibility of overcoming the virus. Remember, approximately 15 percent of people naturally clear the body of the virus at its onset. Anything you can do to increase the odds of this happening is worth considering.

Symptoms reported by people newly-infected with HCV include:

- Flu-like illness
- Diarrhea

2   Ibid.

- Night sweats
- Loss of appetite
- Fever
- Fatigue (mild to severe)
- Indigestion
- Abdominal pain or bloating
- Jaundice (yellowing of the skin and whites of the eyes)
- Nausea

If you have four or more of these symptoms, get tested for Hepatitis C. The earlier you catch it, the better your chances of beating it right away. Obviously, make this same recommendation to friends and family members you care about.

SURVIVAL SECRET

Symptoms felt by MOST patients are not directly connected to liver impairment.

EXTRA-HEPATIC PROBLEMS

Approximately 38 percent of patients past the acute stage, with chronic Hepatitis C will develop some symptoms of at least one extra-hepatic (non-liver) illness. Some of these illnesses and syndromes include neuropathy, lymphoma, fibromyalgia and diabetes. (If you are unfamiliar with any medical terms used in this book, look them up on the internet.) Most extra-hepatic problems appear to be connected to how the immune system responds to the Hepatitis C virus. In addition, a chronic HCV infection seems to be necessary for the development of extra-hepatic problems. Science is beginning to understand the role that HCV has in causing some extra-hepatic "manifestations," but many of the links have yet to be discovered.[3]

The relationship between extra-hepatic conditions and the immune system's response to HCV helps explain why – in many

3   Mayo, Marilyn J. MD; Kaplan, Norman M. MD, Editor; Palmer, Biff F. MD. "Extrahepatic Manifestations of Hepatitis C Infection." The American Journal of the Medical Sciences – Abstract: Volume 325(3) March 2003.

cases – previously asymptomatic patients experience symptoms of neuropathy, fibromyalgia, chronic fatigue syndrome, and others, only after they begin Pegylated Interferon with Ribavirin therapy. The common side effects of Pegylated Interferon with Ribavirin therapy are often identical to the symptoms of Hepatitis C.

Some extra-hepatic complications may develop because your stressed-out liver is placing unusual demands on other systems in the body. In other cases, your body finds it difficult to combat other problems, because it's been weakened by prolonged HCV infection. For these reasons, it's important to take responsibility for staying (or getting) as healthy as possible; visit your primary healthcare provider regularly, make lifestyle and nutrition changes, and avoid drinking alcohol or using any drugs or medicines that are not strictly necessary.

R E C R E A T I O N A L   D R U G   U S E ?

It makes no difference to me whether you contracted HCV from a blood transfusion in 1986 or from a needle you shared with friends in 1999, I am not here to judge (and it certainly didn't make a difference to the virus). But now that you're aware of your disease, it's critical to support your liver and your overall health by discontinuing the use of harmful drugs, tobacco and alcohol – especially alcohol. Alcohol is a toxin that, even in small quantities, places stress on the liver. Look at the word *intoxication:* "toxic" is a key element! The effects you feel during and following intoxication result from how the liver metabolizes and eliminates this toxin.

> *Survivor Story:*
> *"Getting and staying clean and sober, that's the best gift
> I have ever given myself and the knockout punch I've
> delivered to my hep C. If you have hep C and are still
> drinking or otherwise using, please get help from a 12-step
> program or from somewhere else, and give your liver, and
> your life, a chance. You are part of the universe. You have a
> right to live and be happy."*
> *– Alice*

Continuing to share drug equipment increases the likelihood that you'll become infected with another disease, including other forms of Hepatitis, as well as AIDS. And when it comes to cigarette smoking, how can inhaling more than 3,000 chemicals, including dozens of well-known carcinogens, be good for you?

If you're addicted to drugs, including nicotine and/or alcohol, please seek help – from family, friends, support groups, physicians, therapists, or others. If consulting with a Buddhist monk in Tibet helps you kick the habit, then schedule a visit... soon. Do whatever it takes to get that monkey (or monkeys) off your back.

Taking certain prescribed medicines and over-the-counter drugs may also carry risks *(see acetaminophen on page 128, 156)*. Always be sure to check with your doctor.

HEPATITIS C IN PRISONS

According to a press release from the medical journal *Hepatology,* (October 20, 2008) 12 to 31 percent of U.S. prisoners are infected with chronic HCV. Clearly, this is due to highest-risk behaviors among people who end up in prison, such as intravenous drug use.

Many patients' infections are not attended to because guidelines vary from state-to-state regarding treatment. With this high level of prevalence in prisons, all inmates should request testing for HCV, and do their best to protect and support their liver through natural means, whether or not medical treatment is available to them.

SURVIVAL SECRET

The most common genotype in North America is also the hardest to eradicate.

WHY YOUR GENOTYPE MATTERS

I'm revealing my age here, but there used to be a series of TV commercials that continually warned viewers, "All aspirins are not alike!" The same holds true of the Hepatitis C Virus. Again, scientists have identified six different, but related, genetic strains (genotypes) of HCV. Furthermore, these genotypes are divided into 15 subtypes. The classification system works like this: every genotype receives a numeral to distinguish it from the others – for example, genotypes 1, 2, 3, etc. – and the subtypes are assigned a letter (or letters) from the alphabet. For example, the most common genotype and subtype in the United States is "1a", followed by 1b, 2a, 2b and 3a. In Europe, genotype 1b is predominant, followed by 2a, 2b, 2c and 3a. Genotypes 4 and 5 are found almost exclusively in Africa.

Survivor Story:

"I was… unaware until after I started the Interferon therapy and read the materials that came with the medication that genotype 1a is the most resistant to the Interferon combo therapy and has the lowest success rate of reversing the virus."

– James

Why should you care about your virus's genotype and subtype? The answer is simple: the success rate of the conventional treatment for Hepatitis C – a combination of Pegylated Interferon and Ribavirin – differs dramatically, depending on your virus's genetic code. Genotypes 1 and 4 are less responsive to Interferon-based treatment than genotypes 2, 3, 5 and 6. What's more, the duration of standard Interferon-based therapy for genotypes 1 and 4 is 48 weeks, whereas treatment for genotype 2 requires just 24 weeks.

"Cure rates" (sustained viral response) of 75 percent or better are reported in people with genotype 2 within 24 weeks of treatment, compared with rates of less than 50 percent in those with genotype 1 within 48 weeks of treatment, and 65 percent in those with genotype 4 within 48 weeks of treatment. Unfortunately, 70 to 80 percent of Hepatitis C patients in the United States have genotype 1[4].

In summary, 70 to 80 percent of chronically infected Americans have a 50/50 chance (at best) of responding to the standard medical treatment for Hepatitis C. Actually, I believe this number is closer

4   Wikipedia, "Hepatitis C."

to 30 percent. In my opinion, 50 percent is a generous prognosis, because it doesn't count people who don't qualify for the treatment because of contraindications or who can't tolerate treatment because of the potentially debilitating side effects and end up stopping before it is completed.

Plus, as Mark Twain famously said regarding questionable facts – "There are lies, dammed lies, and statistics." He clearly considered the malicious manipulation of statistics the worst offense. And, unfortunately, pharmaceutical companies seem particularly good at this practice. Also, what is currently called a "cure" may simply be remission in many cases before the virus becomes detectable again.

Getting Tested

If you or a loved one has been diagnosed with Hepatitis C, chances are you've already undergone several tests to determine (A) whether you have the disease; (B) the amount of liver damage incurred; and (C) your genotype and viral load. To follow is a summary of the standard tests, as well as my suggestions on discussing "next steps" with your primary healthcare provider.

Liver enzyme tests. These tests measure the quantity of enzymes secreted by the liver. When liver cells die, these enzymes are naturally secreted. There is a normal rate at which liver cells die and are replaced by new ones, and normal enzyme levels in the blood indicate this. When a higher number of cells die, enzyme levels elevate – and this indicates a problem. Abnormally high levels of the enzymes alanine aminotransferase (ALT), aspartate aminotransferase (AST), alkaline phosphatase (ALP), gamma-glutamyl transferase (GGT) and/or 5'nucleotidase (5'N'Tase) in the blood may indicate that your liver has been damaged or is under attack by HCV. It's very important to note, however, that higher-than-normal levels of these enzymes do not necessarily indicate the presence of the Hepatitis C virus. Any number of factors (including other illnesses) can cause abnormal enzyme levels in your blood, with alcohol consumption being the most obvious. Because your liver is the organ most responsible for eliminating waste from the body, any toxins ingested will produce an enzymatic reaction by the liver. Still, these enzyme tests are a good method for determining if something is wrong with your liver.

Liver function tests. These tests measure the levels of proteins manufactured by your liver, comprising albumin, bilirubin and blood-clotting proteins. Low levels of albumin may indicate liver or kidney disease, malnutrition or even a low-protein diet. High levels of bilirubin, a waste product created during the normal death of red blood cells after 90 to 120 days, may be caused by excessive death of red blood cells or because the liver isn't processing the chemical normally, which may indicate liver damage. The blood clotting test (or PT test) measures how quickly your blood clots. If your blood requires more time than normal to clot, this may indicate that your liver, which makes these clotting proteins, isn't producing enough of them.

WHAT OTHER TESTS ARE THERE?

Additional blood tests. A variety of other blood tests offer indirect ways to determine if your liver function may be compromised. But again, these tests – which include everything from measuring your white blood cell count and red blood cell count to the amount of iron and alpha-fetoprotein in your system – simply reveal the possibility of liver problems, not the specific cause(s) of those problems.

Imaging tests. Ultrasound tests, CAT (computed tomography) scans and MRI (magnetic resonance imaging) tests are excellent methods of detecting liver fibrosis (scarring) or cancer, but obviously these devices were not designed to scan for tiny viruses. So, unless you already have significant liver damage, they won't be of much help. Of course, it's never a bad idea to check for liver damage.

Antibody Tests. In my view, these two tests – the EIA (enzyme immunoassay) and RIBA (recombinant immunoblot assay) are the best early detectors of HCV. Why? Because these tests actually "look for" the specific antibodies that are produced by your body when – and only when – the Hepatitis C virus is present.

Hepatitis C RNA Tests. These are the "gold standard" of tests to detect and analyze the presence of HCV. In most cases, your primary healthcare provider – for obvious reasons – won't administer this test until other tests indicate that you may have compromised liver function (after all, you probably wouldn't take your temperature with an oral thermometer unless you first had symptoms of a fever).

As the name suggests, these two tests don't actually "pinpoint" the presence and/or location of HCV, but reveal the presence of the virus by detecting its genetic material – RNA. There are two types of RNA tests: the qualitative RNA test and the quantitative RNA test. The qualitative test simply tells you that – yes or no – HCV is present in your body. The quantitative expanded test more exactly estimates the levels of HCV RNA (ribonucleic acid) in your blood, which is known as your "viral load." Viral load is expressed in international units per milliliter (IU/ml) and can range from 5 IU/ml to millions of IU/ml in those infected with HCV.

SURVIVAL SECRET

You should demand that your doctor tell you what each measurement indicates on your blood test results, and its significance.

Survivor Story:

"Two years ago I never thought I would be around for this long. But, thanks to a lot of lifestyle changing and a couple of good doctors and a little more positive attitude, I'm still here. Today I go for the sixth-month check of my viral load. Last time around they were about 1,000 parts per million. In the very beginning, before the therapy they were at 6 ppm. But a year with the meds and a lot of praying and meditating I am still around. I found it most depressing after six months that the virus came back, but it taught me a few life lessons. One, that you have to try and do what you can. And, two, that there is not any guarantee even when you do what you can."

– Bob

Biopsy. If you've been diagnosed with Hepatitis C (or another liver problem/disease), your physician may ask you to take "the definitive" test to determine the extent of damage (if any) to your liver. Basically, the biopsy requires that your doctor (or another white-lab-coated technician) insert a hollow needle directly through your abdomen and into your liver to retrieve a small "core sample" of tissue. Yes, they use anesthesia to ensure that you don't faint from the pain. On the plus side, the biopsy provides direct evidence of the state of your liver. On the minus side, the procedure is invasive, and in some instances can cause bleeding that will require blood transfusions or surgery to correct; accidental puncture of other vital organs: and/or abdominal infection – not to mention post-procedure pain. Also, this core sample only reflects the condition of your liver exactly where (in the organ) the sample was taken. Your liver may be in much different condition elsewhere.

SURVIVAL SECRET

Dependable biopsy replacements are now becoming more available.

BIOPSY REPLACEMENTS

New Less-Invasive Fibrosis Tests. In the last few years, non-invasive blood tests have been developed to detect liver fibrosis in patients with chronic Hepatitis C. These include FIBROspect II (from Prometheus Laboratories) and HCV-FibroSure (from BioPredictive). There are also APRI, Fib4, and Forns index. The new tests measure biological markers associated with the development of liver fibrosis to help physicians differentiate patients who have no (or mild) liver fibrosis from patients who have significant liver fibrosis. Another test, FibroScan (from Echosens), based on sound, is a new, non-invasive, rapid and reproducible method allowing evaluation of liver fibrosis by measurement of liver stiffness. Although these tests are currently available, they are considered experimental, and your health insurance company may not cover the costs. They are also not necessarily as accurate as biopsy yet. But, if you are completely against having a biopsy, at least you have alternatives to consider.

My "Take" on Testing

As you may have guessed, I'm not a big fan of liver biopsies. Liver biopsies basically require someone to stick a needle into a sick liver; whereas other tests such as FIBROspect II, FibroScan or others mentioned are noninvasive and almost as effective. Early on, I began working with a general practitioner who insisted that I submit to a biopsy. She said, "Do a biopsy. It's no big deal." I said, "Really? Then you won't mind getting in line ahead of me. I'll get my biopsy right after you do."

For some reason, she declined. (Hmmm... I wonder why?)

Survivor Story:

"The biopsy was done in a local hospital in Portland, Oregon. They led me to believe that the surgery would be done via ultrasound, and that most people said it was no big deal. The ultrasound was done by a nurse that used it only to make an ink dot on my right side between two ribs. She and the radiologist practiced breathing with me as I lay there on the table. When the time came, the radiologist counted one, two, three... and told me to hold my breath. He shot the "harpoon" through my side, asked me if I was all right, looked at the [sample] that he extracted from my side, and said, "Wow, that was definitely a big sample." I still couldn't breathe. I began to cry, as it hurt like being shot... The tears were falling down my cheeks, and I couldn't speak to let them know how much pain I was in. Apparently, the mechanism malfunctioned, and got a bunch of "white and gray" tissue along with the liver biopsy. I was admitted to the hospital and given morphine. I was finally able to take full breaths 48 hours later. I will NEVER undergo another liver biopsy under any circumstances."
– Nicole

Risks aside, the main reason I'm not in favor of biopsies is because, for most Hepatitis C patients, a biopsy will have little or no impact on the suggested course of treatment – i.e., on "next steps." For asymptomatic Hepatitis C patients, knowing your viral load, genotype, subtype and enzyme levels is much more important for determining treatment options, than it is for determining your level of fibrosis. I'm not suggesting that fibrosis levels aren't important – they are – but since these can be estimated with the new blood tests, why have someone stick a big needle into your side?

When I was first diagnosed with Hepatitis C, I felt very healthy (and I still feel quite healthy, partially thanks to my natural regime, I'm sure). I knew my genotype (1a), and my enzyme levels weren't dramatically elevated, so I thought a biopsy was irrelevant. The results wouldn't have changed what I was going to do, so I didn't want to subject my liver to the procedure. I'd already decided to try the more natural or holistic route to maintaining my health.

Keep in mind, however, that I decided not to undergo the conventional treatment because my genotype is the least responsive to Pegylated Interferon with Ribavirin therapy, and for various other personal reasons. You, on the other hand, may decide that the conventional approach is right for you, and PLEASE don't think I'm trying to change your mind.

My point is not to dissuade you from getting a biopsy or using Pegylated Interferon with Ribavirin therapy, or to persuade you to undertake alternative tests and treatments. I just want you to be informed, which is what the rest of this book is about. I'd also like to caution you against accepting your physician's word – or anyone's word, including mine – as gospel.

SURVIVAL SECRET

Work WITH your doctors, because they work FOR you.

Western medical practitioners are not bad people, but most are very conservative people. Frankly, I don't blame them. Given the escalating cost of malpractice insurance, it makes little sense for doctors to risk their careers and reputations on unconventional tests and medicines. They are also very busy. That's why most doctors stick with the tried and true. It's why they generally insist on biopsies and Pegylated Interferon with Ribavirin therapy. These are considered the medical "gold standard" of care in cases of Hepatitis C.

So, it is up to you to get smart, ask questions, make better lifestyle choices and let your doctor know what you are doing and what you want to do about your condition at each and every stage or visit.

SURVIVAL SECRET

Viral load is apparently not directly related to possible or actual degree of liver damage being caused by the virus.

VIRAL LOAD RELEVANCE

A "high" viral load does not mean one person is sicker than someone else with a "low" viral load. Part of this secret is that viral load fluctuates up and down, sometimes quite dramatically. So take your viral load with a large grain of salt. It's not an accurate measure of how sick you are. I've known people with viral loads in the 300 million IU/ml range who could beat up Superman, and others who couldn't get out of bed with viral loads of just 20,000 IU/ml. Viral load is just one way of estimating the virus population in your system.

One more point regarding viral load: very high viral load (5 million IU/ml and beyond) in genotype 1 patients apparently makes the virus harder to defeat with current medical therapies.

As a fellow Hepatitis C survivor, your health and well-being are important to me. Many people have helped me, and I want to help you. If you have any questions about anything in this chapter, feel free to email me at Ralph@HepCSurvival.com. New information about this disease is becoming available regularly. You can to stay up-to-date by signing up for important email notifications (and a FREE 6-part "survival" e-course) at http://www.HepCSurvival.com. This way, I can keep you informed with the latest news, and help you get the most out of this book. You'll also find a multitude of important resources through the website, including my analysis and commentary on new information as I discover it.

CHAPTER 2

Is Medical Treatment Right for You?

SURVIVAL SECRET

Worth repeating:
Far more of us will die WITH
this disease than from it.

In my opinion, especially for patients with genotype 1 like myself, one key to being a survivor is to stay as healthy as possible until a real cure, or a much more effective (and less debilitating) treatment is discovered. Remember, the United States Centers for Disease Control (CDC) estimates that 70 to 80 percent of North Americans with Hepatitis C have genotype 1, which is the most resistant to today's standard therapy – Interferon and Ribavirin. For people with genotype 2 or 3, there's a much greater likelihood that this therapy will work and, frankly, if I'd been diagnosed with genotype 2 or 3, I might have given it serious consideration (except for those potentially horrific side effects).

Survivor Story:

"*I feel okay mostly except trouble sleeping and, since I have genotype 1a, I decided not to go on treatment yet until there is something more effective and less toxic. My doctor three years ago said I can afford to wait after getting a biopsy (which was not painful). I think he said it was mild so far. I don't like the idea of those side effects that treatment can cause. I guess I still have enough energy for now, but I worry since one of my friends has recently died from Hep C and I also found out that two other people I once knew have it, and one of them has died also. Plus, I have met other people recently who are on the waiting list for a liver transplant.*"

　　　　　　– Betty

SURVIVAL SECRET

Research into this disease (and treatment) is quite extensive and ongoing.

Always ask your healthcare provider for the latest information (or look it up yourself). Even some things you find in this book could be outdated by the time you read them. So, don't hesitate to dig deeper. To stay updated, sign up for email alerts at *http://www. HepCSurvival.com*. That way, you can stay informed about any new and relevant information, and benefit from all my ongoing legwork and research. I'm constantly doing the research for myself anyway, so you may as well benefit, too.

INTERFERON AND RIBAVIRIN

Interferon is a protein (specifically a cytokine) naturally produced by your cells to fight viral infections. Pegylated Interferon alpha 2a and Pegylated Interferon 2b (don't ask me about the names) are the mainstay of the current combination treatment. Basically, these drugs boost your immune system in fighting off the Hepatitis C virus. How? Well, scientists aren't quite sure, but they do know that the drug helps a significant number of patients. They also don't know why it's more effective in destroying some HCV genotypes than others. When they do understand more, that will probably presage a cure for Hepatitis C – whether or not the cure involves Interferon.

Ribavirin is an anti-viral drug that, by itself, has no effect on Hepatitis C Virus (HCV). In combination with Pegylated Interferon, however, it enhances your ability to fight the virus. Again, nobody knows why.

If you opt for combination therapy, you'll need to self-inject Pegylated Interferon every week, and take Ribavirin in pill form every day. Thankfully, both of the pharmaceutical companies making these drugs have devised easy ways to administer injections, using either pre-filled syringes or injection pens.

In 1989, criteria for patient acceptance regarding Interferon therapy were published, partially determined by the National Institutes for Health. Criteria included length of time a patient had had the disease, confirmation that the patient had HCV infection, and lack of severe liver injury.

Here is a full list of criteria:
- Elevated ALT for at least six months
- Hemoglobin less than 11g per deciliter
- White blood cell count of less than 3,000 per microliter, as well as polymorphonuclear leucocytes less than 1,500 per microliter
- Liver biopsy verifying diagnosis of chronic hepatitis
- Albumin more than 3g per deciliter
- Bilirubin less than 4mg per deciliter
- Prothrombin time less than 3 seconds beyond control
- No signs of hepatic failure (demonstrating current compensated liver disease)
- Platelet count above 70,000 per microliter.

Also, those patients with the best results appear to be:

- Asian or Caucasian
- Under 50 years of age
- Female
- HCV genotypes 2 or 3
- Of healthy weight
- Lacking fatty liver (steatosis)
- Suffering minimal liver damage
- Non-diabetic
- Demonstrating a healthy immune system

As stated, genotype is now also taken into consideration because certain genotypes respond more successfully to treatment. Viral genotypes 2 and 3 apparently respond quickly and well to current medical treatment. According to a review article published in the February 2009 issue of the medical journal *Hepatology*, the success rate for 24-week treatment of genotypes 2 and 3 is upwards of 70 to 82 percent. Remembering what Mark Twain said, that's a claim of half the treatment time for genotype 1, with about double the success rate.

SURVIVAL SECRET

African-Americans have a significantly lower success rate with current therapies than Caucasians, and people of Asian descent have a significantly higher rate of success.

Some studies also suggest African-Americans have a much slower progression of the disease. The data regarding African and Asian response disparities indicates a genetic component to treatment response. Be sure to get the latest information from your doctor specific to your circumstance.

There are currently five varieties of Interferon medication with a positive effect against HCV. Two of these are Pegylated, which means they are processed to remain in your bloodstream longer and be released slower and more consistently over a longer more sustained period of time. Only two companies make these Pegylated forms, Roche (Pegasys) and Schering-Plough (Pegintron).

As already stated, these Interferons are most commonly used in combination with Ribavirin (together known as combo therapy among Hepatitis C patients). By combining Ribavirin with Interferon the sustained antiviral response of Interferon therapy is greatly enhanced. This is why combo therapy is considered the best form of medical treatment for Hepatitis C. Again, the standard treatment duration is 48 weeks for genotype 1, and 24 weeks for genotype 2 and 3. The treatment goal is to clear the virus from your body, which is called a sustained virological response, or SVR. One source states that an SVR of 40 to 50 percent is achieved in HCV Type 1 patients (which I still believe is well-inflated) and 70 to 80 percent for types 2 or 3 (also likely inflated).

SURVIVAL SECRET

To prepare the injection site prior to taking Interferon, press hard with your thumb for a minute or two and it tends to desensitize the area.

OVER-THE-COUNTER PAIN RELIEF DURING TREATMENT

You are going to be injecting yourself regularly and anything you can do to alleviate the discomfort is welcome. Ibuprophen is considered one of the best over-the-counter medicines for pain. Naproxen Sodium is also very good, and lasts longer. You might also want to try applying ice to the area for a minute or two to achieve a comparable numbing effect. Some people have few or gentle side effects, most experience more than just a little discomfort.

SOME SIDE EFFECTS OF TREATMENT

Common side effects of Interferon include flu-like symptoms (chills, muscle aches, headaches, weakness, tiredness, for example.) Other effects might be nausea or diarrhea and weight loss. Fatigue can be quite severe and may require treatment with drugs. Before trying anti-fatigue drugs, learn your limits and avoid overextending yourself. When you plan your time, allow blocks for napping or relaxation. Also, let people know you have energy limits and learn to say "no" more often.

Still other effects include depression, moodiness, impaired concentration (or what many call "brain fog"). Depression occurs more frequently in people who have experienced it before, but that is not always the case. Antidepressants are often prescribed for people during therapy. Those with a history of severe depression may find themselves ineligible for treatment because of clinical concerns regarding their depression.

Being cranky and irritable during treatment is quite common. Thyroid, kidney and autoimmune symptoms can occur, as well. Also, hair loss, thyroid disease, severe platelet drop, or increase of underlying autoimmune diseases like IBS, rheumatoid, arthritis and systemic lupus is also possible, although rare.

You may also become more prone to infection due to the therapy, so even dental surgery is discouraged. One key area of concern is white and red blood cell counts, along with platelets; which is a key reason regular blood tests are given during treatment. As stated earlier, Natalie Cole received a kidney transplant in 2009 because of the damage this treatment for Hepatitis C did to her kidneys.

Common side effects of Ribavirin include:

- *Anemia:* this is related to the breakdown of red blood cells but is also made worse by the drug's suppression of bone marrow to create new red blood cells. This anemia can be so severe that it can affect the heart and other organs. Therefore, people at risk of cardiovascular problems are often given a cardiac stress test before therapy.

- *Rash:* located anywhere around the body, this side effect is very common. Reduction of Ribavirin usually helps.
- *Mouth and throat issues:* taste distortion, chronic cough and mouth pain are all attributed to the drug's effect on the mucous membranes of the mouth and throat and can by reduced by a reduction of the drug.

Due to these three common side effects alone, approximately 26 percent of patients require dose reduction during therapy. To underscore its potential danger, the FDA requires a "Black Box" warning on this treatment.

I've communicated with thousands of Hepatitis C survivors, many of whom have tried combination therapy. The minority experienced minimal side effects, while most found the side effects to be very uncomfortable and more than a little debilitating. Most people intensely regretted the experience. (Keep in mind, however, that many people contacting me didn't have a successful course of treatment – people the doctors call "non-responders.") It is estimated that there are up to 300,000 non-responders out there now, just trying to stay as healthy as possible until another therapy arrives. If you know one, you may want to recommend this book to them because it provides hope, and information on alternatives they can use to support and protect their liver in the meantime.

Here are some representative stories of reactions to medical treatment submitted to me by other Hepatitis C survivors:

Survivor Story:

"My husband started on the combined treatment, shots of Interferon weekly and Ribavirin every day. He was a walking zombie – throwing up for the first few weeks and just feeling miserable. He had NO energy and was in a lot of muscular pain. It was like he was shooting poison into himself every week. After about six months, he came to me, and said he just couldn't do it any more. He needed to stop the treatment and get to a place in his life when he could try again.

*He went to his doctor, who wasn't very happy about
stopping. [The doctor] asked that he get checked every six
months so if his numbers went back up, they would be on
top of it... His levels have been NORMAL ever since."*
– Savannah

Survivor Story:

"*During treatment, I had to let go of practically my entire
social life. I had been active in a mom's club, and usually
got together with friends once or twice a month, usually
for dinner after work or a Saturday afternoon of museums
or hiking. I had to stop all of those activities – I was just
too tired. Even though I was taking a nap almost every
afternoon, I was heading to bed at 9:00 p.m. every night,
totally exhausted (and often nauseated). Even weekends
were mostly devoid of activities. I needed the weekends to
recharge and get ready for the next week's work. I found
that if I did anything social on the weekend, I would be
tired the whole next week. It just wasn't worth it. My
insurance (and my family's) is through my work, so not
working was not an option. My life consisted of work and
home. Period.*

*Luckily, I had good insurance, and it covered just
about all of the treatment. I had to spend $30/month for
the Rebetol [a brand name of Ribavirin], and nothing for
the Peg-Interferon. The side effects from the Rebetol were
pretty bad. I understood that if a person had ever suffered
from depression that these drugs were not for them, but
I have always been a cheerful sort, so I wasn't worried.
But several times near the end of treatment, I would hear
myself say the meanest things to my kids and it just killed
me. I would hear the hurtful words come out of my mouth
and see the looks on their faces, and I wanted to take the
words back so badly, but it was already out and there was
nothing I could do. I completed a six-month course of*

treatment. The virus was way down after the first month, and by the time I was finished, it was undetectable. My new, treatment-aggressive doctor wanted me to go another three months, but I just couldn't face it."
   – Sharon

Survivor Story:

"After I was on the combo therapy of Interferon and Ribavirin, I developed neuropathy in my feet. I started out on Neurontin, but now I'm on Oxycontin twice a day. I also got real fat... and developed diabetes about a year after. Depression is the one thing that doesn't go away. I was taking a number of antidepressants including Zoloft, which in my opinion works the best."
   – Mike

SURVIVAL SECRET

Statins may improve sustained viral response when used in conjunction with conventional combination therapy.

This statin information is according to a report published in the medical journal *Hepatology* in July 2006, regarding the work of M. Ikeda, A. Ken-ichi, M. Yamada, and others. Of course, statins may cause other problems, so do your homework.

ASK YOUR DOCTOR WHAT ELSE MIGHT HELP

When it comes to genotype 1, a gastroenterologist I know called Interferon "a drug looking for a disease to cure." And in his opinion, Hepatitis C (especially genotype 1a) is NOT that disease.

As already stated, the drug companies claim combination therapy offers a 50 percent chance of achieving a sustained virologic response for genotype 1, meaning the virus is undetectable for at least six months after treatment. But as my earlier Mark Twain quote pointed out, statistics can be twisted and convoluted. Based on my reading, nothing has convinced me that Pegylated Interferon and Ribavirin therapy achieves more than a 30 percent success rate for people with genotype 1 (my guesstimate is based on taking 100 people with HCV Genotype 1, putting them in a room and counting those who could start therapy based on existing contraindications, those who could complete therapy, and those who would complete therapy AND achieve a sustained viral response – as they call the current "cure"). And yet, 70 to 90 percent of patients experience negative effects.

A simple cost/benefit analysis says that if something has a 30 percent chance of working and (at minimum) a 70 percent chance of making you feel like garbage, there has to be a better way. Another factor in my personal decision to pursue alternative therapies is that I was (and am) feeling very good. I'm not in dire straits. My liver enzyme levels aren't highly elevated, and I don't have extra-hepatic symptoms. For these reasons, my gastroenterologist and I decided there was nothing wrong with pursuing alternative treatments. He knows I'm doing natural therapy, and he monitors my condition every six months, tests my blood, and determines if I'm remaining stable.

So far, the strategy has paid off. I'm not trying to scare you away from the standard treatment, but I think you should understand both the benefits and drawbacks. Always weigh the pros and cons before pursuing one treatment versus another. It's YOUR body!

SURVIVAL SECRET

If you can't afford therapy (and you meet certain criteria) you may qualify for free medication.

AFFORDING THERAPY

Each of the two suppliers of treatment offer free drug programs (though you still need to pay for certain elements including doctors and tests) Contact Schering-Plough or Roche directly for information about their respective programs for those who otherwise could not afford therapy. Or, go to Partnership for Prescription Assistance – *http://www.pparx.org,* or Needy Meds – *http://www.needymeds.org.*

DOING NOTHING (MORE OR LESS)

As previously stated, according to the CDC, 20 to 30 percent of people with chronic Hepatitis C will eventually suffer from potentially life-threatening liver complications. Flip that statistic over, however, and it means that 70 to 80 percent will not. Keep this in mind if/when your doctor says, "You've got chronic Hepatitis C. It's a deadly disease, and we really should treat it with combination therapy – right away!" As I said earlier, doing nothing is an option. By "doing nothing," however, I do not mean absolutely nothing, or (worse) continuing to indulge in bad habits.

Doing nothing does not mean:
- Continuing to drink alcohol.
- Using recreational drugs.
- Smoking cigarettes.
- Eating a typical junk food diet and growing obese.
- Leading a sedentary life.

Doing nothing simply means that you're not pursuing a mode of treatment – conventional or alternative – designed to actively support and improve liver function or reduce your viral load. It means taking care of yourself in a more healthful way. It may involve lifestyle changes, including drinking more water, eating more nutritious foods, exercising more often, and finding non-chemical ways to reduce stress.

Survivor Story:

"I had two friends who were infected, and as 15-year-olds, we tried intravenous drugs. Truth is, I tried [them] maybe four times... but that didn't stop me from getting infected... It only takes once. I know a few others who HAVE to be infected, as they did it with the same group, but – of course – since they have no symptoms, they either refuse to believe it or would rather not quit drinking and bury their heads in the sand... My girlfriend is an alcoholic, and now has cirrhosis. She still drinks, so I know she is not long for this world, but there's nothing I can do. I've tried, and so has her family."
  – Libby

You may be doing nothing to specifically kill the virus and support your liver, but you're doing something to address the health of your body, right? If you're not, you certainly should be!

What convinced me to avoid conventional treatments in favor of alternative treatments, is I took into account my overall condition, lifestyle, health, as well as my genotype. You can do the same. Right?

What About More Advanced Cases?

On the other hand, if you're among the minority of patients with advanced fibrosis or cirrhosis, doing nothing is not an option. These are serious conditions that require aggressive medical intervention. Depending on the degree to which your condition has progressed, the intervention isn't necessarily combination therapy, especially since some doctors consider cirrhosis to be irreversible, but it could include certain herbs (including the phytosome form of milk thistle). Some complementary and alternative medical (CAM) therapists believe it's possible to slow, stop and possibly reverse cirrhosis with herbs and other natural interventions. But, cirrhosis is a very serious medical condition, even in its early stages. That's why it's important to get informed, get more than one medical opinion – remember, M.D. does not stand for "medical deity" (they are not gods) – and investigate your treatment alternatives, medical and /or otherwise.

Survivor Story:

"I got my hep C from sharing a needle when I was using. I hope my story will help. The most important thing is to have a positive attitude and remember that it's not a death sentence."
        – Howard

It's well within your power to live a long, productive life with Hepatitis C and die at age 95 in your sleep from something else. You may be able to live healthier and better through natural means, which I'll discuss in the following chapters. And don't forget that new, potentially more effective and body-friendlier therapies are on the horizon (or so the pharmaceutical companies claim). Actually, finding a more effective and less-toxic treatment could be such a profitable business for them, that a myriad of companies are scrambling to come up with something better. Their greed may work to our advantage in the long run. How poetic.

Whether or not you choose medical treatment, I urge you to consider the nutritional supplements, herbal preparations, as well as dietary and lifestyle changes recommended throughout this book. Protecting and supporting your liver when you have a chronic and potentially deadly disease, is not just a "nice" idea, it is an imperative.

As a fellow Hepatitis C survivor, your health and well-being are important to me. Many people have helped me, and I want to help you. If you have any questions about anything in this chapter, feel free to email me at *Ralph@HepCSurvival.com*. New information about this disease is becoming available regularly. You can to stay up-to-date by signing up for important email notifications (and a FREE 6-part "survival" e-course) at *http://www.HepCSurvival.com*. This way, I can keep you informed with the latest news, and help you get the most out of this book. You'll also find a multitude of important resources through the website, including my analysis and commentary on new information as I discover it.

CHAPTER 3

Are Any Natural Products Proven To Help?

SURVIVAL SECRET

Natural remedies may
have real benefits.

In a landmark paper, it was estimated that 34 percent of the general population has used complementary and alternative medicine (CAM)[5] – a figure that rocked many people in the conventional medical establishment – and that number is increasing exponentially. It's easily over 50 percent by now. Complementary and alternative therapies are usually defined as those not widely taught in medical schools, not generally used in hospitals, and not typically reimbursed by medical insurance companies. But this situation is rapidly changing. It's estimated that more than 50 medical schools in the United States now offer courses in CAM, with some acknowledging the huge popularity of these therapies by establishing centers for integrative medicine (which combine CAM and conventional medical treatments).[6]

5   Eisenberg DM. "Advising patients who seek alternative medical therapies." Ann Intern Med 1997, 127: 61-69.
6   Bass, Nathan M., MD, Ph.D. Is There Any Use for Nontraditional or Alternative Therapies in Patients with Chronic Liver Disease? Current Gastroenterology Reports 1999, 1:50-56

COMPLEMENTARY/ALTERNATIVE MEDICINE

As reported by Dr. Nathan M. Bass:

There has been a substantial increase in the use of so-called complementary and alternative therapies by patients with liver disease. Although many such modalities are available, herbal therapies are the most popular, and of these remedies, silymarin extracted from the milk thistle is most widely subscribed to as a remedy for liver diseases. Available evidence points to a potential, but unproven, benefit for this as well as other therapies based on free-radical scavenger or antioxidant principles in treating patients with liver disease. These therapies deserve further investigation through experimental studies and well-controlled clinical trials... As practitioners educating and treating patients with liver disease, we are obliged to be informed about popular alternative therapies, understanding of our patients' need to be partners in their care, and open-minded to the possibility that some benefit may come from some therapies currently regarded as "alternative". We need to be effective and tolerant in learning about which alternative treatments our patients are taking, so that we can monitor their effects if any and counsel appropriately against those that may cause harm.

I should mention that NONE of the natural products described in this chapter has been specifically proven to fight the Hepatitis C virus (HCV) itself, but they all have demonstrated benefits in supporting and protecting liver function and health. This isn't to say they don't help fight HCV – only that science doesn't yet know. Much research has yet to be done, and in the meantime, any product or treatment that can protect and support liver function is certainly worth investigating.

There are possibly hundreds of substances (supplements, herbs, foods, formulas, for example) that could be good for your liver. The trick is to find those with the most "proof" of effectiveness and safety at the lowest cost, *while never sacrificing quality for price.* Otherwise, if you tried to take "everything" that might help you could be popping pills and drinking potions all day long and go broke in the process. What I've done for you is narrow down a list of what I believe can give the greatest benefit at the least cost. This assessment is now based on decades of research.

Survivor Story:

"I feel lucky that my PCP (primary care practitioner), gyno and my liver doctor are all pretty open to alternative therapies. I've questioned them all about it, and my gyno says he thinks there is a lot to be offered through herbs and vitamins, but that they don't do enough research on it, and won't until they know they can make a buck, and I feel the same way... I, of course, buy milk thistle... I have a vitamin regimen of C, E and B complex, along with selenium (off and on), and alpha lipoic acid (off and on)..."
– Libby

Milk Thistle – The Superior Phytosome Form

Milk thistle (as is most effectively and affordably found in MegaThistle), with the scientific name *"Silybum marianum"*, is a plant native to the Mediterranean that now grows wild in Europe, California and Australia. Used in Europe since the 16th century as a treatment for liver disease and jaundice, the active ingredient of the herb is silymarin, which is found in the fruit.

After being diagnosed with Hepatitis C, I consulted with naturopaths, homeopaths, clinical nutritionists, and holistic MDs (among others). One of the first products I began taking was milk thistle extract because so much was written about its successful centuries-long use around the world for liver ailments. Also, every holistic practitioner I spoke with recommended it without reservation. There was no other herb that had such an impressive reputation as milk thistle for liver support and protection.

At the time, I took the best 80 percent standardized extract I could find, and milk thistle has been the mainstay of my regimen ever since. However, I've made one critical change regarding this product. I now only use and recommend the phytosome form as found in MegaThistle.

SURVIVAL SECRET

Many studies show milk thistle's beneficial effects on the liver, but the best effects are not found in just any off-the-shelf brand...

...which could contain much less active ingredient than your liver needs. You ought to choose the form in MegaThistle for the greatest liver protection, support and regeneration – you can find MegaThistle at the lowest price through *http://www.megathistle.com.*

In the February 1999 issue of the *International Journal of Integrative Medicine,* I came across an article about milk thistle written by a naturopathic physician. Most of the article was a rehash of information I already knew, but in one paragraph the author mentioned a clinical study on a superior form of milk thistle that was shown to be dramatically more absorbable. She stressed that one of the only shortcomings of regular standardized milk thistle extract was extremely poor absorption. But by combining the extract with phosphatidylcholine (PC), researchers achieved eight- to ten-times more absorption. And eight- to ten-times more absorption means up to 1,000% more protection for your liver.

At first, in my naïve simplicity, I thought all I had to do was take my milk thistle along with lecithin (which contains high levels of PC) in order to deliver more milk thistle to my liver. Researching further, I discovered that the process was much more sophisticated than that. The developers actually bound one molecule from the milk thistle extract to two molecules of PC. The resulting patented compound is called Siliphos™ (also known as Silybin Phytosome), which is much more like a medicine, and less like a supplement. I think of it as a super-charged delivery system of highly effective liver protection. Your body soaks up PC like a sponge soaks up water. The milk thistle extract goes along for the ride through your bloodstream to where it does the most good, your liver.

SURVIVAL SECRET

Because of the way it is manufactured, MegaThistle is much more like a medicine than a mere herbal extract.

WATER HOSE OR FIRE HOSE, YOUR CHOICE

What impressed me the most about the phytosome form of milk thistle were the published clinical studies showing the dramatic superiority regarding absorption of this product over any other form of milk thistle. There are very few nutritional supplements that have this kind of scientific validation to back up their claims of safety and effectiveness. You can find many of these studies at *http://www.megathistle.com/studies*. With this in mind, why would you choose any other form?

Doing more research, I found that Siliphos (or Silybin Phytosome) was available as a finished product through Enzymatic Therapy (a highly respected mainstream nutritional supplement company), so I started buying it at the health food store. At the same time, I came upon clinical studies that had been carried out on the product. One study conducted with hepatitis patients showed the median helpful dosage was 240mg taken three times per day.

The bottle of Enzymatic Therapy's supplement contains 60 capsules of just 120mg. The recommendation on the bottle called for one to two capsules per day. This was nowhere near what the study recommended. To attain the study dosage, I needed to take six capsules per day, which meant one bottle only lasted ten days. That came to three bottles per month at $21 per bottle, for a total of $63 per month. I felt that was a bit expensive, even for such a powerful product.

I knew this overpricing put the product out of range for most people, so I researched the possibility of offering the formula directly on the internet to cut out distributor and retailer costs and keep the price more reasonable. I saw this as a way to help others. Eventually,

I decided to go directly to consumers through the internet, which allowed me to offer the lowest price available. Back then, I was able to reduce the cost to as low as $25 per bottle for the same amount of product that cost $63 through Enzymatic Therapy, and even more through other suppliers. My approach delivered dramatic savings to Hepatitis C survivors everywhere, and convinced me that I was right to move forward, to help others get this product easily and affordably, so we named the product and went live with it. Since launching in August 2000, that product has helped thousands of people get the best milk thistle product.

Since its introduction, over 250,000 bottles have been purchased by smart, informed, survivors like you. I subsequently came out with a higher-potency version based on the highest potency tested in the scientific studies. That product was one-third stronger (360mg per capsule instead of 240mg).

I've recently developed a new product based on this dosage, and it's called **MegaThistle.** This new product, even at the higher potency, can still be purchased for much less than any comparable product offered elsewhere. You can get much more in-depth information regarding its proven ability to **most effectively** help you protect and support your liver at *http://www.megathistle.com.*

Survivor Story:

"My biopsy results revealed little to no inflammation, no scarring and no fibrosis. My specialist felt I would be a good candidate for combination treatment. Looking back I would never have chosen the drugs for therapy. I did not realize then that for my genotype the chances of non-detection after treatment were slim. I was so sick and tired through much of the treatment. The Interferon caused other problems like an overactive thyroid which I now take medication for. I currently take the milk thistle formulation (ed: as found in MegaThistle). I figure if I need to take milk thistle, it might as well be the one that is most absorbed into my body, drink green tea, and take a multivitamin without iron. I am starting to take a new vitamin for the

fatigue I experience to see if it helps. I also drink plenty of
water and get regular exercise."
  – Janice

MILK THISTLE BENEFITS

I have no doubt that milk thistle is beneficial based on the clinical studies I've read about milk thistle in general and the more powerful phytosome formula in particular, although I must admit I am biased, having done so much research during product development (and, using it myself for over ten years). Both in vivo and in vitro, milk thistle extract has been scientifically proven to support, protect and regenerate healthy liver cells. In many cases, elevated enzyme levels are reduced.

Even when enzyme levels are unaffected by milk thistle, fibrosis appears to be slowed considerably, according to a study cited in *Gastroenterology Journal* by Dr. Detlef Schuppan. Dr. Schuppan is considered one of the world's leading experts on milk thistle and liver disease. This study was entitled: *Antifibrotic Effect of Silymarin in Rat Secondary Biliary Fibrosis is Mediated by Downregulation of Procollagen Alpha1(I) and TIMP-1.* These results were published in the *Journal of Hepatology* in September of 2001.

Survivor Story:

"I started making a list of things to do before I died... I didn't want to die regretting the things I didn't do. I knew I could not change things I had already done, but I knew I could do things I'd always wanted to. After being on the milk thistle formulation (ed: as found in MegaThistle) for 18 months, I had another biopsy and viral load done. MIRACLE! I had regressed back to Stage 2 [fibrosis] and my viral load was down by two-thirds! The doctor urged me to go back on Interferon, stating there were other drugs available now to help the side effects and they were having improved response. He said I was in prime condition to tolerate it. I declined. The success rate was not high enough to risk losing my life, and I could not envision being on that medicine again and living through it."
  – Peggy

SURVIVAL SECRET

Herbs are used more like drugs in Europe and Asia, where they are prescribed by doctors.

U.S. DOCTORS ARE ALSO TAKING HERBS SERIOUSLY

In Germany, and other countries, herbal preparations are actually prescribed by doctors. The German *Commission E* (the equivalent of our FDA) was tasked with scientifically validating and rating herbal preparations as drugs. They found milk thistle to be helpful for liver conditions, as well as being nontoxic and having no known drug interactions or contraindications. The German *Commission E Monographs* (considered by knowledgeable physicians to be the bible of herbal effectiveness and safety) consequently classify milk thistle as an approved herb.

Under the category of "Uses", the Commission E Monographs state: "Toxic liver damage; for supportive treatment in chronic inflammatory liver disease and hepatic cirrhosis."
Under the category "Actions" it says, "The therapeutic activity of silymarin is based on two sites or mechanisms of action: (a) it alters the structure of the outer cell membrane of the hepatocytes in such a way as to prevent penetration of the liver toxin into the interior of the cell; (b) it stimulates the action of nucleolar polymerase A, resulting in an increase in ribosomal protein synthesis, and thus stimulates the regenerative ability of the liver and the formation of new hepatocytes." This means it helps to protect and regenerate healthy liver cells.

Survivor Story:

"In a way, this virus has been a gift. It forces me to be aware of the choices I make. I make sure that I eat right, exercise, and get plenty of rest. At first, I was taking all kinds of vitamins and herbs, but have now narrowed it down to

*those I feel are most important. I take a good food-based
multi-vitamin without iron, extra vitamins C and E, along
with... R-alpha lipoic acid. One of the most important herbs
I take is the phytosome form of milk thistle (ed: as found in
MegaThistle). I also take a product called Liv.52. Although I
still get tired sometimes, I feel so much better overall. I can't
even remember the last time I had a cold. I do believe there
is a better treatment on the way, maybe even a cure in the
near future. Until then, I take good care of myself and live
my life to the fullest."*
  – Denise

Many people ask if they will see or feel a difference when taking
milk thistle products. The fact is, some people do, and some don't.
Elevated enzyme levels may be reduced (indicating a reduction in the
liver cells dying on a daily basis), but this is not true in all cases. Yet,
as Dr. Schuppan pointed out, this doesn't mean the herb isn't helping
to protect and support healthy liver function and inhibit fibrosis.

Some people report feeling fewer aches and pains, more energy,
less brain fog, and a reduction in other symptoms. Because this varies
from person to person, no promises or even suggestions can be made
about how it may affect any individual. Look at it this way, people
don't feel a difference when they take cholesterol-reducing drugs, but
that doesn't mean the drugs aren't doing their job saving lives.

Survivor Story:
*"My PCP referred me to a gastroenterologist who I am
comfortable with and who has never tried to push me
into treatment. He was very upfront and told me about
treatment and that I should do a lot of research before
making my decision. I decided I would NOT put that
poison in my body unless I HAD to. I know there is a
chance it could cure me and I could do fine with minimal
side effects, but I am not willing to take the chance of
living in misery and coming out worse than when I started.
My friend, Tim, suggested I check out the phytosome form*

(ed: as found in MegaThistle) and my doctor agreed that
while he can't say it would help, but that in his opinion, it
couldn't hurt."
  – Hal

As stated earlier, the key difference between regular (or standardized) milk thistle and the phytosome form is absorption. When considering the absorption of the phytosome-based MegaThistle, take all the studies about milk thistle benefits and multiply by up to 10, because that's how much more reaches your liver (and how much less goes into your toilet). This also makes MegaThistle a much greater value based on how much more of its medicinal properties actually gets to your liver cells.

PLEASE DON'T EAT THE PLANT

I occasionally encounter websites, blogs and individuals extolling the supposed benefits of ingesting dried milk thistle in its natural form or as a tea (actually, the active ingredients in milk thistle are not even water soluble, which means the tea is all but useless).

For the sake of kindness, I'll assume these individuals believe that the benefits of milk thistle – like those of many vitamins – are best obtained from the original vegetation, rather than taking pills. Okay, that may be true of some herbs, but it's absolutely not the case with milk thistle – and most other liver protection/support herbs.

SURVIVAL SECRET

Standardized herbal extracts are generally stronger than simple dry herbs. Standardization allows for higher and consistent levels of active ingredients.

How Does an Herb Become A Medicine?

Milk thistle's active extract (silymarin) is derived from the seeds and is found in much lower concentrations in the unprocessed plant. When you buy 80 percent standardized milk thistle, the seeds have been processed and purified to contain 80 percent silymarin. When you buy the phytosome form, it has been purified even further. Silymarin is made up of several bioflavonoids. The three most active ones are silybin (sometimes spelled silibin, silybinin or silbinin), silychristin, and silydianin.

Silybin makes up 50 to 60 percent of silymarin and has been proven to have the most beneficial effect on the liver. In fact, all of silymarin's beneficial effects can be directly attributed to silybin. This is why MegaThistle is made with pure silybin, because it is the most active and beneficial constituent for anyone with liver concerns.

Historically, the process of isolating the most active constituent of a plant or substance is a common practice in pharmacology. Many medicines were initially derived from natural sources. A good example would be the drug Digitalis. This is a heart medicine derived from the foxglove plant. It's isolated and purified to be used as a medicine. There would be no additional value in eating an entire Foxglove plant (and it would taste terrible). The full benefit is contained in the Digitalis.

Another example would be aspirin. Originally isolated from the bark of willow trees, salicylic acid has been proven to help alleviate certain aches and pains. While you could chew on a bunch of willow bark and get even more elements than just the active ingredient, all you really need is the salicylic acid to get rid of your headache. And it would take quite a lot of bark chewing to provide the equivalent of two aspirin tablets.

Now consider milk thistle. Silybin has been shown to be the most active beneficial constituent of the plant for your liver. The company, Indena S.p.A., which produces the superior patented formula, Siliphos (or Silybin Phytosome), isolates the silybin, and binds it to phosphatidylcholine in a proprietary process that increases absorption by up to 1,000 percent. (see charts at *http:// www.megathistle.com.)* So not only are you getting a super-charged delivery system, the system delivers the most valuable and beneficial constituent of the milk thistle plant by using another substance, phosphatidylcholine, that is also vital to a healthier liver (you can read more about that later).

In my opinion, if you are going to take just one supplement to treat your Hepatitis C infection, it should be milk thistle. And, if you are going to bother taking milk thistle, then it should be MegaThistle for maximum benefit versus cost. As already stated, MegaThistle is made with the phytosome form of milk thistle. Just looking at the published scientific studies should convince you this is your best bet to protect and support healthy liver cells. (For a list of research studies on milk thistle, please go to *http://www.pubmed.com.)* This is the U.S. National Library of Medicine online. In the search box at the top of the page just put in milk thistle or silymarin, or silybin, or silybinin, or silibin or silibinin, or siliphos, or silybin phytosome, or IdB 1016, or silipide – all related to the same substance I am recommending most highly to you here – and notice the hundreds of published studies you get, overall.) To make it easier for you to research, just go to *http:// www.megathistle.com/studies.*

L I V . 5 2
This is a traditional Indian Ayurvedic medicine currently marketed under several names, including LiverCare.

SURVIVAL SECRET

I believe Liv.52 is most helpful for people exposed to multiple toxins, especially alcohol.

ARE YOU REGULARLY EXPOSED TO TOXINS?
Liv.52 might help. The Liv.52 formula contains the following ingredients:

- Capers *(Capparis spinosa)* – a well-documented liver stimulant and protector that improves the functional efficiency of the liver.
- Wild chicory *(Cichorium intybus)* – a powerful hepatic stimulant that increases bile secretion, acts on liver glycogen and promotes digestion.
- Black nightshade *(Solanum nigrum)* – which promotes liver and kidney health, and has shown liver-protective activity in cases of toxicity induced by drugs and chemicals.
- Arjuna *(Terminalia arjuna)* – a general tonic for the heart and liver that regulates the biosynthesis of hepatic cholesterol.
- Yarrow *(Achillea millefolium)* – a stimulative tonic for the liver that promotes effective elimination of toxins.
- Tamarisk *(Tamarix gallica)* – a hepatic stimulant and digestive that has been shown to have a salutary effect on the liver.

The combination of these medicinal plants has been widely used and researched in India for over 30 years. Further, because the formula has been widely tested in animals and used clinically for some time, its lack of toxicity has been well documented. Although Liv.52 appears to be beneficial in treating liver disease and may play a role as an antioxidant herbal preparation in supporting the liver function of people with Hepatitis C, there is no clinical evidence (that is, no human studies) that Liv.52 has an anti-viral effect on the Hepatitis C virus itself, or that it can prevent or treat cirrhosis.[7]

Like all herbal remedies, Liv.52 works through a combination of mechanisms that yield a broad variety of health benefits. In this case, most of the mechanisms can be placed into two categories: ingredients with hepatostimulant (liver stimulant) properties or those with hepatoprotective (liver protective) properties.

In addition to toxicity and experimental studies to gauge the safety and mode of action of Liv.52, clinical studies have also been conducted on humans to assess and confirm the efficacy of Liv.52. Altogether, more than 300 studies have been conducted over five decades, making Liv.52 one of the most studied and tested herbal

7   Patrick, Lyn, ND. *"Products Marketed to People with Hepatitis C."* Hepatitis C Choices, Caring Ambassadors Program, 2004.

products in the world. Because of the broad range of benefits, many clinical investigators throughout the world have proven the value of Liv.52 in a range of situations, including its ability to promote healthy levels of liver enzymes.[8]

Liver enzyme levels are the most common measure for determining whether the liver is functioning properly, and Liv.52 has been shown to help maintain normal levels on various liver function tests. This result is associated with normalized liver enzyme levels and stimulation of the natural hepatic cell repair process.

Finally, Liv.52 has also been studied in relation to its mechanism for protecting against certain hepatotoxic substances. In the case of alcohol, for example, the protection mechanism centers on rapid elimination of acetaldehyde, a metabolite of alcohol.[9] Put simply, Liv.52 has been proven as a powerful formula for helping the liver to detoxify the body, as well as to protect and even repair liver cells.

Survivor Story:

"I also was not aware, until after I started the Interferon therapy and read the materials that came with the medication, that genotype 1a is the most resistant to the Interferon combo therapy and has the lowest success rate of reversing the virus. I started therapy and two weeks later was in the hospital due to my heart going into atrial fibrillation (A-fib). Since I have never had heart problems, and one of the side effects of the Interferon therapy is hyperthyroidism (which can cause A-fib), it was determined that in all likelihood, the therapy had caused my heart to go into A-fib. I immediately stopped the therapy and am now dealing with getting my heart back into rhythm. I am sure that for some people the Interferon can reverse the virus; I just want to inform everyone that you need to thoroughly investigate what you are doing before you agree to go on this potent medication. Examine your lifestyle and determine if you

8   "A study of serum glycolytic enzymes in relation to Liv.52." Med. And Surg. 1986; (4):9.
9   "The effect of Liv.52 on absorption and metabolism of ethanol." Eur. J. Clin. Pharmacol. 1991; (40): 189.

can make more changes in your diet, exercise, alcohol intake, etc, before resorting to Interferon. Hopefully, in the future, something better will come along for us. Until then, I will continue down the non-toxic road of silybin phytosome (ed: as found in MegaThistle), Liv.52, no alcohol, healthy diet and exercise. I hope my story helps."
– Richard

HONSO BRAND SHO-SAIKO-TO (FORMULA H09)

Sho-saiko-to is one of many herbal formulas found in the traditional Japanese medicine chest (Kampo), which was originally derived from traditional Chinese medicine (TCM). As of 1996, the Japanese Ministry of Health and Welfare has approved 148 different Kampo formulas for reimbursement under its national health insurance plan, and 75 percent of Japanese physicians currently use Kampo in combination with conventional medical prescriptions. The Honso brand is the one available here in the USA. Sho-saiko-to has been prescribed over 1.5 million times by Japanese doctors for all forms of hepatitis and liver concerns.

The key difference between Japanese Sho-saiko-to and the liver-support formula used in traditional Chinese medicine is that the Japanese formula has been standardized with regard to the amount and proportion of ingredients. The herbal components of Sho-saiko-to are: water-based extracts of bupleurum root, pinellia tuber, scutellaria root, ginseng, jujube, licorice and ginger.

Two major chemicals from scutellaria (baicalin and baicalein) are strong inhibitors of lipid (fat) peroxidation. In tests with rats that had been given toxins, the extract of scutellaria prevented damage to the cell membranes of the liver and restored mitochondrial function. This increases the levels of superoxide dismutase and gluatathione produced by the liver, both of which are important for proper liver function, protection and support. Sho-saiko-to has also been observed to possess anti-tumor properties and may contain agents that protect the liver against fibrosis. Clinical research on the formula's efficacy as an anti-viral agent is still rudimentary, but the data are promising.

One more important point about Sho-saiko-to; there is a new, untested form that is encapsulated (called SST). The original form is a powder that you mix with water, and the 1.5 million Japanese prescriptions mentioned earlier were filled with the powder form. In my mind this would certainly increase absorption, and for that reason I would NOT recommend the capsule form. Let's face it; if I'm going to take a product, I want the form that's been prescribed over one million times for liver concerns. With Sho-saiko-to, that is the powdered form (available only through health care providers). You can learn more about the powder form at *http:// www.HepCSurvival.com/H09.*

PRECAUTIONS

Unlike Siliphos® (or silybin phytosome), and Liv.52, Sho-saiko-to should not be taken by people with certain medical conditions or taking certain drugs. Sho-saiko-to should not be taken:

- If you have an existing lung impairment such as asthma, or if you're a cigarette smoker.
- If you are currently undergoing treatment with Interferon.
- If you have a platelet disorder.
- If you suffer from hypertension.
- If you are taking other products containing licorice.
- If you are pregnant or nursing.
- In addition, a small percentage of individuals are sensitive to bupleurum, the primary herb in the formula. If the following conditions develop or worsen while taking Sho-saiko-to, discontinue its use:
  - Migraine headaches.
  - Very high blood pressure (systolic over 180 mmHg).
  - Epistaxis (nose bleeds).

As stated above, the original dosage form of Sho-saiko-to is available only through healthcare providers. Because I am a licensed provider in New York I can give you access to this powerful remedy. You can find out more information regarding this at *http://www.HepCSurvival.com/H09.*

SOME LIVER-TOXIC HERBS TO AVOID

This section would not be complete without a list of known liver toxic herbs that you must avoid:

- Borage
- Chaparral
- Comfrey
- European mistletoe
- Germander
- Golden ragwort
- Groundsel
- Heliotropium
- Hemp agrimony
- Kava
- Margosa
- Pennyroyal oil
- Sassafras
- Senna
- Skullcap
- Tansy ragwort
- Uva ursi
- Valerian

SURVIVAL SECRET

Just because something is "natural" doesn't mean it is safe.

Remember, the deadly poison cyanide is naturally-derived, too. You need to be educated AND selective.

As a fellow Hepatitis C survivor, your health and well-being are important to me. Many people have helped me, and I want to help you. If you have any questions about anything in this chapter, feel free to email me at *Ralph@HepCSurvival.com.* New information about this disease is becoming available regularly. You can to stay up-to-date by signing up for important email notifications (and a FREE 6-part "survival" e-course) at *http://www.HepCSurvival.com.* This way, I can keep you informed with the latest news, and help you get the most out of this book. You'll also find a multitude of important resources through the website, including my analysis and commentary on new information as I discover it.

CHAPTER 4

Do You Know the Best Natural / Alternative Treatments?

Although "the jury is still out" on whether the herbs and herbal formulas described in the last chapter directly affect the Hepatitis C virus, there is overwhelming evidence that they provide significant benefits when it comes to protecting, supporting and even restoring liver structure and function. With regard to the alternative treatments summarized in this particular chapter, however, there tends to be less evidence – aside from anecdotal evidence (or stories) – to back up claims for their effectiveness. Of course, the success of many of today's best medicines was first recognized at the anecdotal level before research and testing demonstrated that they worked. At minimum, the treatments in this chapter meet the second criteria set by Hippocrates in his famous saying: "As to diseases, make a habit of two things – to help, or at least to do no harm."

WHAT ABOUT NATUROPATHIC DOCTORS?

In my opinion and experience there are good and bad doctors of every kind. I like the fact that naturopathic physicians have a variety of natural approaches to work with. Unfortunately, some of those approaches are on my "dubious" list. However, in the hands of a naturopath, using a variety of modalities, these approaches certainly can do no harm and may even do more good than if practiced or approached individually.

Also, the approaches most commonly used by Naturopathic doctors will do much less harm than most pharmaceuticals. (Did you know there are an estimated 106,000 deaths per year from PROPERLY PRESCRIBED pharmaceuticals, not to mention those that are mis-prescribed?)

SURVIVAL SECRET
Our bodies have a powerful, innate instinct for self-healing.

WHAT IS NATUROPATHY BASED ON?

Here is a description of naturopathy from The American Association of Naturopathic Physicians:

"Naturopathic medicine is based on the belief that the human body has an innate healing ability. Naturopathic doctors (NDs) teach their patients to use diet, exercise, lifestyle changes and cutting edge natural therapies to enhance their bodies' ability to ward off and combat disease. NDs view the patient as a complex, interrelated system (a whole person), not as a clogged artery or a tumor. Naturopathic physicians craft comprehensive treatment plans that blend the best of modern medical science and traditional natural medical approaches to not only treat disease, but to also restore health."

WHAT ARE THEIR RULES?

Naturopathic physicians base their practice on six timeless principles founded on medical tradition and scientific evidence:

Let nature heal. Our bodies have such a powerful, innate instinct for self-healing. By finding and removing the barriers to this self-healing – such as poor diet or unhealthy habits – naturopathic physicians can nurture this process.

Identify and treat causes. Naturopathic physicians understand that symptoms will only return unless the root illness is addressed. Rather than cover up symptoms, they seek to find and treat the cause of these symptoms.

First, do no harm. Naturopathic physicians follow three precepts to ensure their patients' safety: 1) Use low-risk procedures and healing compounds – such as dietary supplements, herbal extracts and acupuncture – with few or no side effects. 2) When possible, do not suppress symptoms, which are the body's efforts to self-heal. For example, the body may cook up a fever in reaction to a bacterial infection. Fever creates an inhospitable environment for the harmful bacteria, thereby destroying it. Of course, the naturopathic physician would not allow the fever to get dangerously high. 3) Customize each diagnosis and treatment plan to fit each patient. We all heal in different ways and the naturopathic physician respects our differences.

Educate patients. Naturopathic medicine believes that doctors must be educators, as well as physicians. That's why naturopathic physicians teach their patients how to eat, exercise, relax and nurture themselves physically and emotionally. They also encourage self-responsibility and work closely with each patient.

Treat the whole person. We each have a unique physical, mental, emotional, genetic, environmental, social, sexual and spiritual makeup. The naturopathic physician knows that all these factors affect our health. That's why he or she includes them in a carefully tailored treatment strategy.

Prevent illness. "An ounce of prevention is worth a pound of cure" has never been truer. Proactive medicine saves money, pain, misery and lives. That's why naturopathic physicians evaluate risk factors, heredity and vulnerability to disease. By getting treatment for greater wellness, we're less likely to need treatment for future illness.

NATUROPATHY PRACTITIONER TRAINING

Which schools are approved and where are Naturopathic doctors allowed to practice? You should know that in the United States and Canada, the designation of Naturopathic Doctor (ND) may be awarded after completion of a four year program of study at an accredited Naturopathic medical school that includes the study of basic medical sciences as well as natural remedies and medical care. The scope of practice varies widely between jurisdictions, and naturopaths in unregulated jurisdictions may use the Naturopathic Doctor designation or other titles regardless of level of education. A 2004 survey determined the most commonly prescribed naturopathic therapeutics in Washington State and Connecticut were botanical medicines, vitamins, minerals, homeopathy, and allergy treatments.

In the U.S. there are five accredited Naturopathic colleges (you don't want a naturopathic doctor who did not attend one of these):
• Bastyr University, Seattle, WA
• University of Bridgeport College of Naturopathic Medicine (UBCNM), Bridgeport, CT
• Southwest College of Naturopathic Medicine & Health Sciences (SCNM), Phoenix, AZ
• National College of Natural Medicine (NCNM), Portland, OR
• National University of Health Sciences, Chicago, IL

U.S. jurisdictions that currently regulate or license naturopathy include: Alaska, Arizona, California, Connecticut, District of Columbia, Hawaii, Idaho, Kansas, Maine, Minnesota, Montana, New Hampshire, Oregon, Puerto Rico, US Virgin Islands, Utah, Vermont, and Washington. Additionally, Florida and Virginia license the practice of naturopathy under a "grandfather" clause.

U.S. jurisdictions that permit access to prescription drugs: Arizona, California, District of Columbia, Idaho, Kansas, Maine, Montana, New Hampshire, Oregon, Utah, Vermont, and Washington.

U.S. jurisdictions that permit minor surgery: Arizona, District of Columbia, Idaho, Kansas, Maine, Montana, Oregon, Utah, Vermont, and Washington.

U.S. jurisdictions which specifically prohibit naturopathy: South Carolina, and Tennessee.

In Canada there are two Naturopathic Colleges (you don't want a naturopathic doctor who did not attend one of these):

- Boucher Institute of Naturopathic Medicine (BINM), Vancouver, British Columbia
- Canadian College of Naturopathic Medicine (CCNM), Toronto, Ontario

There are five Canadian provinces which license naturopathic doctors: British Columbia, Manitoba, Nova Scotia, Ontario, and Saskatchewan. British Columbia has regulated naturopathic medicine since 1936 and is the only Canadian province that allows certified ND's to prescribe pharmaceuticals and perform minor surgeries. A common problem with naturopathy, is that even where it is legally recognized, it is not always covered by health insurance.

TRADITIONAL CHINESE MEDICINE (INCLUDING ACUPUNCTURE)

Five thousand years old, traditional Chinese medicine (TCM) currently treats more than a billion people in China and Southeast Asia, including the roughly 30 million Chinese suffering from Hepatitis C.

SURVIVAL SECRET

Traditional Chinese Medicine may help, if you find a good practitioner.

According to well-known TCM practitioner Qin Cai Zhang, MD, this "vital health and healing system... is based on harmony or balance. A healthy person is in complete balance, both with him or herself and with nature." Traditional Chinese medicine theory states that disease is a deviation from balance, and the purpose of treatment is to restore it. TCM focuses on maintaining health rather than managing disease. TCM is an empirical medicine, meaning it was developed mainly through clinical observations. It is a logical system that summarizes the results of clinical observation and experience to instruct further practice.

Survivor Story:

"I drink lots of water and herb teas (dandelion tea, licorice root tea and milk thistle tea) and I take lots of vitamins and herbs. I did have acupuncture, and that was good..."
    – Estes

TCM has developed unique diagnostic and therapeutic methods such as tongue diagnosis, pulse reading, herbal formulas, acupuncture, tui na (Chinese massage), and qigong. TCM treats patients holistically – that is, as a whole, rather than treating individual parts. This ancient medical system is continuously developing.

One of the two key principles underpinning TCM is "qi" (also spelled chi), which is your life-force energy. According to TCM, when qi is in balance, all is well. When qi is out of balance, you are susceptible to disease. The other underlying principle is that of yin and yang – two halves of the same whole – which must be in balance to preserve overall good health.

TCM IS "IFFY" FOR HEPATITIS C VIRUS

TCM offers different treatments for Hepatitis C and/or its symptoms, including acupuncture, acupressure and moxibustion (the burning of Chinese herbs on various points of the body to warm energy channels). TCM also uses exercises such as T'ai Chi and Qigong, as well as meditation and breathing exercises. Outside of acupuncture, the most popular treatments are custom-tailored herbal formulations. For example, the Chinese equivalent of Sho-saiko-to is known as xiao-chai-hu-tang. It contains the same ingredients as Sho-saiko-to, but TCM physicians add, subtract or adjust dosages based upon each patient's unique needs. Since each person's imbalance has a unique presentation, there are a variety of herbal formulas that a TCM physician may use to help those with Hepatitis C. It is NOT a one-size-fits-all medicine. And I know of no one who has been cured of Hepatitis C by TCM.

Beverly's experience with a noted TCM practitioner is fairly typical:

Survivor Story:

"My internet search for herbal treatments led me to a traditional Chinese doctor who was also a hepatologist, immunologist and herbalist. I began treatment in June 2004. I began the herbal treatment on faith, since the ingredients in the treatment will not be disclosed to you. I rely on the results of the hepatic function panel blood tests that I have taken periodically to monitor the reduction in my ALT levels, and the other factors as explained to me by the doctor, to determine if the cost of the herbal treatment is a worthwhile investment in my health and the fight to curb future liver damage resulting from the Hepatitis C virus.
– Beverly

Survivor Story:

"I discontinued the use of the other herbs that I had been taking, and began his herbal medicine of chewable tablets and herbal pills. While it's too soon to know if I will be able to discontinue the herbal treatment, as some patients have, or at least continue on a long-term maintenance dose of a half or quarter of my current dosage, I can attest to the fact that my ALT levels are decreasing towards the

normal range of 2-40. My doctor's goal is to maintain an
ALT level of 20. My [previous] ALT levels were 201 and
252 before the herbal treatments. After beginning this
herbal medication in June 2004, my ALT levels decreased
to 93, and then 74."
　　　　　– Alice

TCM claims many anecdotal successes such as this, which isn't surprising, since the most popular herbal formulation (xiao-chai-hu-tang) contains the same ingredients as Sho-saiko-to – albeit not in standardized amounts and proportions.

The problems I have with TCM are:

- The proprietary herb formulations are available only from TCM practitioners because they are "customized" for each individual patient. Unlike Siliphos (or silybin phytosome) formulations, Liv.52 or Sho-saiko-to, you can't buy TCM products anywhere else.
- You don't know precisely what's in these formulations – unless you take a sample to your local CSI crime lab.
- The overall practice of TCM is as much art as science, leaving you dependent on the reputation and alleged skills of each TCM physician.

SOME PEOPLE SWEAR BY TCM

Then again, I've spoken with many people who've used traditional Chinese medicine and done very well with it. However, if you apply a cost/benefit analysis, the most important thing to remember is that TCM physicians are not curing you. They don't claim they can cure you. Their approach is to correct "imbalances". They may be fortifying your liver and enhancing your overall health, but there are many other ways – and often much less expensive ones – to do this (as I've already shown).

Does this mean there's not a place for TCM? No, but I believe that most TCM practitioner-provided herbal formulations are overpriced.

The cost difference between the Phytosome® form of milk thistle found in MegaThistle, for example, and a secret herbal formulation from a TCM doctor is often as high as $1,200 per month! Obviously, price is not the only consideration. If it works, continue using it – if you can afford to. For myself, however, I'd rather use that extra $1,200 per month (if I even had it to spare) for other things!

I spoke with one woman whose husband had Hepatitis C, and she wanted to find something cheaper than the TCM formula he'd been using. I suggested a number of products from my personal "A-List" of supplements I take, but her husband didn't respond as well to them. So, they returned to their TCM doctor and his high-priced formulas. That's fine. At least they experimented.

Some TCM practices, particularly massage and acupuncture – may address extra-hepatic symptoms. Muscle joint pains and fatigue may all be relieved by those. Traditional Chinese medicine is obviously accomplishing something, since it's been used for thousands of years by millions of people. It's gone through millennia of trial and error. However, because TCM is usually custom-tailored to the individual, it is unfortunately nearly impossible to measure objectively the results in a larger population.

AYURVEDIC MEDICINE

The word Ayurveda means "life" (ayush) and "science" or "knowledge" (veda). Like TCM, Ayurvedic medicine is a complex and ancient compendium of theories, observed wisdom and medical practices that treats patients in a holistic fashion – body, mind and spirit. To determine the best treatments for a particular ailment, Ayurvedic physicians attempt to diagnose everything about the person and his environment.

Ayurveda calls the life-force energy the "prana," which is concentrated in seven different energy centers in the body, called the "chakras." In Ayurvedic medicine, every human being is characterized based on his or her combination of the three "doshas" (or energy patterns). These are:

- *Vata.* Composed of space and air, this is the subtle energy associated with all voluntary and involuntary movement in the body, governing breathing, blinking, muscle and tissue movement, as well as heartbeat. Vata has a tendency to expand indefinitely, and disturb the nervous activity or the vital forces in the body.
- *Pitta.* Composed of fire and water, it is responsible for all digestive and metabolic activities, governing body temperature, complexion, visual perception, hunger and thirst. In a balanced state, pitta promotes intelligence, understanding and courage. Out of balance, pitta produces insomnia, burning sensations, inflammation, infection, anger and hatred. Pitta is the humor involved in liver disorders.
- *Kapha.* Composed of water and earth, it provides the strength and stability for holding body tissues together. It is the watery aspect of the body. In balance, kapha is responsible for wisdom, patience and memory. Out of balance, kapha causes looseness of the limbs, lethargy, greed and a generalized sluggishness (or hypo-activity).[10]

WHAT DO AYURVEDIC DOCTORS SAY?

According to Doctors Shri K. Mishra and Sivaramaprasad Vinjamury, "The treatment of liver disorders usually involves a combination of herbs, bodywork, dietary advice, lifestyle changes, yoga and meditation. It is important to follow a specific diet and curtail excessive activities. Depending on the person's physical state, treatment begins with a mild laxative, which is either limited to the start of treatment or taken daily. If the person is unable to tolerate the laxative, it is stopped and treatment proceeds to the next step. After cleansing, oral medications are given two- or three-times daily. These medications can be herbal concoctions, powders, pills, fermented syrups and/or herbs processed in clarified butter (ghee). The dosage, form, and combination of medications are

10   Mishra, Shri K., MD, MS, Bharathi Ravi BAMS (Ayurveda) and Vinjamury, Sivaramaprasad, MD. "Ayurvedic Medicine" Hepatitis C Choices, Caring Ambassadors Program, 2004

selected depending upon the patient's constitution, stage of disease, and physical condition. Only an experienced Ayurvedic healthcare provider can make appropriate medication recommendations...

"Medicinal plants have been used for the management of liver diseases by Ayurvedic and other traditional healers for thousands of years. Numerous plants and herbal formulations containing several botanicals are reported to have liver protective properties. Nearly 150 chemicals from 101 different plants have been claimed to have liver protecting activity. Most studies on hepatoprotective plants are carried out using chemically-induced liver damage in rodents. Several plants have been reported as hepatoprotective in animals by investigators from India during the last decade."

While it may be tempting to regard Ayurveda (and TCM for that matter) as being based on the kind of medieval superstitions that once formed the European barber-surgeon's medical universe, there's no denying that some patients have benefited from Ayurvedic treatments. Keep in mind, the Liv.52 formula was developed from traditional Ayurvedic medicine – just as Japanese Kampo represents a more modern effort to purify and combine the ingredients in various traditional Chinese herbal concoctions. Both Liv.52 and Sho-saiko-to are more like medicines than the traditional herbal remedies on which they're based, but they are still based on these ancient medical traditions. You can learn more about each of these remedies at *http://www.HepCSurvival.com.*

As a fellow Hepatitis C survivor, your health and well-being are important to me. Many people have helped me, and I want to help you. If you have any questions about anything in this chapter, feel free to email me at *Ralph@HepCSurvival.com.* New information about this disease is becoming available regularly. You can to stay up-to-date by signing up for important email notifications (and a FREE 6-part "survival" e-course) at *http://www.HepCSurvival.com.* This way, I can keep you informed with the latest news, and help you get the most out of this book. You'll also find a multitude of important resources through the website, including my analysis and commentary on new information as I discover it.

Which Alternatives May Not Be Worthwhile?

Cost/benefit analysis is important with alternative therapies.

You have to realize that virtually every vitamin and herb company has some sort of liver-care formula. They are all interested in capitalizing on the market of people like you and me who have liver concerns. Just because they suggest or claim that their product is good for your liver does not mean it is the right or best product for you. My rule of thumb when examining such claims and/or products is "when in doubt, leave it out."

There may be hundreds of natural substances that are good for your liver, but none have been proven to be "cures", and most are not helpful in regard to dealing the Hepatitis C virus itself. You need to choose carefully those natural substances that may do the most good at protecting and supporting your liver. One way this can be achieved by following the recommendations made in this book.

Survivor Story:

"I have been to many different professionals – from various gastroenterologists, herbalists, naturopaths, homeopaths and a doctor whose practice is limited to Integrative Medicine... If one is financially capable of paying for all [this], one probably could benefit. I have gained some knowledge from it all... and I carried on as long as possible, but the end result was that I had to declare bankruptcy."
   – Rita

SURVIVOR, BE SELECTIVE

A certain company in Canada, for example, is selling a product in the U.S. that it's not even allowed to market in Canada because of the inflated and unsubstantiated claims it is making. All the company's proof regarding benefits to the liver consisted of foreign studies that aren't even recognized by the Western medical establishment (you certainly won't find them at the National Library of Medicine). Worse still, this company recommends that Hepatitis patients take its product for six months and no other supplement or herb. Why is that? So customers won't feel as bad about spending around $100 per month on this questionable product? Where is patient choice here? What danger would there be in also taking milk thistle, N-acetyl cysteine (NAC), R-lipoic acid, selenium or even a good multi-vitamin without iron?

Another well-known company in the liver supplement arena was fined $60,000 by the Federal Trade Commission for making unsubstantiated claims about its products. This is unfortunate. Someone deficient in any of the elements included in this product might have realized some real benefits.

Survivor Story:

"Mine is truly a story of trial and error. I first learned of the virus in 1997. My viral load was over 1 million. So, I began my journey like so many of us, "no clue, and scared".
I was told by my doctor to take as much milk thistle as

I could afford, not to drink alcohol, and minimize stress and negativity as much as possible. After my first biopsy I had stage 3 fibrosis, after my second I had stage 1. Thanks for all the support from fellow survivors, and keep smiling. There are a host of other things you can do without injections, but everyone is different. There are new drugs coming. Keep the faith."
    – Rick

Whole grains, fruits and vegetables are excellent sources of nutrition and dietary fiber, and eating them certainly promotes good health. So too, most of the products reviewed in this chapter offer genuine health benefits. But none of these products have been shown to arrest or reverse the damage caused by Hepatitis C, with the possible exception of certain Traditional Chinese Medicine (TCM) formulations (for this reason, I haven't included TCM in this chapter, though I consider most TCM custom formulations to be outrageously expensive).

ENERGY HEALING

If you've seen the movies *"What the Bleep Do We Know"* or *"Quantum Communication"* or even *"The Secret"* you understand there is a belief that quantum physics (à la Einstein and his pals) proves that everything is energy. What appears solid to us is just a collection of atoms and smaller particles/waves moving and vibrating at different frequencies. A subset of this belief is that human consciousness (and certain practices/interventions) can effect this subatomic energy. This is the basis for most claims of the possibilities for energy healing (and even attracting abundance).

Based on this science of quantum physics there are many approaches to healing that could be considered "energy healing".

IS THIS REALLY SCIENCE?

Although there is science to support a variety of energy healing modalities, as well as the power of our thoughts and emotions on our healing, this is not an exact science and requires your involvement to truly get lasting results.

While this stuff gets kind of "woo-woo" really fast, you should really watch one or more of the movies above before you count out the theory altogether. You may even be able to get them at your local library. Then you can decide if you want to explore further.

I don't know how much different modalities of energy healing can help Hepatitis C patients, but I've never heard of anyone hurt by these approaches. Some might be very helpful for symptom management (like acupuncture, for instance). However, I would not use any of them exclusively as my entire approach to dealing with Hepatitis C. Especially without also considering exercise, nutrition, supplementation, herbology, stress management, and many other of the fundamentals mentioned in this book.

WHAT ARE SOME OF THE MODALITIES?

Well, anyone who calls themselves a hands-on or distance "healer" is on some level using energy medicine. There are also many other modalities that could be considered to be, on some level, energy healing.

A non-comprehensive list would include:
- Reiki
- Healing Touch
- Therapeutic Touch
- EFT (Emotional Field Therapy)
- TFT (Thought Field Therapy)
- Polarity Therapy
- Qi Gong
- Huna
- Shamanic Rituals
- Ho'oponopono-Hawaiian Healing
- Acupuncture
- Acupressure
- Homeopathy
- Distance healing
- Prayer

- Sound Healing
- Sacred Geometry
- Breathe Work
- Reflexology
- Massage
- Flower Essences Therapy
- Aromatherapy
- Crystal Healing

With energy healing, the shifts can be subtle and yet profound. In many cases the shifts can cause the body to go into a detox state or into what is commonly called a healing crisis. These states may be uncomfortable and yet can do the body a world of good. Energy Healing also is the most likely type of healing that will bring up uncomfortable emotions that have been stored at a cellular level. With the right practitioner, who is understanding and compassionate you can make great progress through these subtle shifts and the emotional breakthroughs that can be achieved with energy healing.

My Opinion on Energy Healing

We've all heard of people being healed miraculously by someone or some thing. There are certain people who swear by certain "healers". In this world, anything is possible. If you want to try a healer who comes highly recommended to you, I see no reason not to (except, perhaps, cost). Again, I consider myself to be an open-minded skeptic. I believe there is much we do not know, and that we do not know what we don't know.

However, be forewarned, with no regulation and/or ways to verify the credentials or efficacy of any of these practices or practitioners you need to watch carefully for scam artists. I set my B.S. meter on high while checking out any of these possibilities for myself.

You might consider also learning to tune in and recognize the intuitive messages that can help guide you through this path or any of the other methods as well. Nothing is for everyone and so it's very important that you learn to identify what is best for you and to use discernment and your intuition to do so.

THYMUS – I THINK NOT

The thymus is a gland involved in the regulation of the body's immune response. Thymus extract products consist of peptides taken from the thymus glands of cows or calves (mad-cow, anyone?) that are sold as dietary supplements. Often, these products carry claims of boosting the immune system to combat diseases such as Hepatitis C. (These over-the-counter thymus supplements should not be confused with the prescription drug thymosin alpha-1.)

According to a 2003 Research Report issued by the National Center for Complementary and Alternative Medicine (NCAM) of the National Institutes of Health, "There has been little testing of bovine thymus extract for treatment of Hepatitis C. A small clinical trial of a product called Complete Thymic Formula, which contains bovine thymus extracts along with vitamins, herbs, minerals and enzymes, did not find the product beneficial for Hepatitis C patients who had not responded previously to Interferon therapy. However, this small study does not provide sufficient evidence to draw firm conclusions about either Complete Thymic Formula or thymus extracts in general.

> *"In the study of Complete Thymic Formula, one adverse event was reported: a patient developed thrombocytopenia, a drop in the number of platelet cells in the blood. The patient recovered after treatment was stopped. In general, no adverse effects from thymus extracts have been reported. However, since thymus extracts are derived from animals, there can be concern related to possible contamination from diseased animal parts. Accordingly, people on immunosuppressive drugs or who have suppressed immune systems, such as transplant recipients or persons with HIV/AIDS, should use caution about thymus extracts and consult with their healthcare provider."*

Frozen thymus is actively promoted to Hepatitis C survivors, especially on one website which I deem questionable at best. By the way, one month's supply of these products typically costs about $250.

And that's a lot of money in my book, especially for something that can't even remotely claim to be a cure.

Moreover, I believe that the rationale behind taking thymus – that it enhances your immune system's ability to fight the virus – is of questionable value. Many extra-hepatic effects of Hepatitis C mimic chronic fatigue or fibromyalgia. You may experience fatigue, body aches, headaches and "foggy brain." None of these symptoms occurs because your liver is impaired to any great degree. In fact, some scientists attribute these symptoms to a hyperactive immune system – an auto-immune response.

HYPING YOUR IMMUNE SYSTEM

It's my feeling that "hyping" your immune system may actually exacerbate some extra-hepatic symptoms. For example, the reason that your liver swells (the inflammation that puts the "itis" into hepatitis) is due to your body's immune reaction. The virus doesn't cause the inflammation; it's your body's attempts to destroy the virus that causes the inflammation. So, if you overly upgrade your immune reaction, you might make your symptoms worse. You want to balance and support your immune system, not knock it into overdrive.

It's also important to note that, while fighting the virus, your body creates scar tissue (fibrosis) in the areas where the "battles" are taking place. Nobody knows why this happens, but the evidence suggests that it's true.

So, if the makers of raw thymus and thymus formulations are claiming that their products will boost my immune system, I'm not sure that's what I want. Although it's important to monitor what the virus is doing to your liver, it's just as important to determine what your body's "war on the virus" is also doing to your liver, not to mention your overall health.

One famous example of an immune response that killed millions of victims occurred during the 1918 influenza pandemic. Physicians and researchers noted that the youngest and most physically fit people died in the greatest numbers. Why? Because their immune systems overreacted to the "intruder" (the influenza virus) and decided to pursue the "total-wipe-out option."

EUROCEL ™

Eurocel is a proprietary herbal formula containing Patrina villosa, Artemesia argyi, Ixeris dentata, Allium tuberosum, Capsella bursa pastoris and Schisandra fructus (say all that three times, fast). Although these herbs have been used historically in TCM formulations for the treatment of liver ailments, one problem with the Eurocel formula (like many TCM formulas) is that the Korean manufacturer will not disclose the exact quantities of each ingredient. On one website, unpublished research is cited attesting to the formula's efficacy in reducing the viral loads of 10 patients in South Korea, but no "outsider" (to my knowledge) has ever seen this study. In addition, the product is quite expensive: I've seen it priced as high as $150 for a 30-day supply.

Not long after I learned about Eurocel, I tried it for a year under the supervision of my gastroenterologist, who monitored my condition through blood tests every three months. I must admit that my viral load decreased consistently, but I wasn't crazy about the cost. Yet, I know of some patients who swear by it and would not do without it. If you can afford to take it on a regular ongoing basis, shop around for the best price and give it a try for three months. I know one patient who sees a huge positive benefit of the product dramatically lowering her enzyme levels (and making her feel better), unlike any other natural formula she has tried. She simply refuses to do without it.

LIVERITE ™

Liverite is a nutritional supplement containing B complex vitamins, phospholipids, cysteine and bovine liver hydrolysate (cow liver that has been broken down by enzymes). Although studies examining the effects of the supplement on liver cells have appeared in European and Japanese medical journals, human studies have not shown any clear benefit in treating Hepatitis C.

Liverite is a mainstream, over-the-counter product that you can find in many drug stores, including your local Rite-Aid. I assessed it some time ago, and it seemed to me that the ingredients could help compensate for certain deficiencies. For example, the B vitamins, including thiamin, are proven to be good for the liver. However, there seemed to be little (if any) evidence that the product would be of much benefit unless you happen to be deficient in B vitamins. Liverite is not expensive, so price is not really the issue. It doesn't make this chapter not because it's overpriced, but because it's over-valued for those who do not have those deficiencies.

TRANSFER FACTORS/COLOSTRUM

Colostrum is the pre-milk fluid produced by female mammals during the first 48 hours following birth. It's thought to possess immune boosting properties essential for the baby who, in the womb, has no immune system of its own. (If the baby did have its own immune system, the mother's immune system would detect it as "foreign matter" and destroy it.) Colostrum is rich in vitamins, minerals, and protein, but its most important functions are to provide the baby with disease-fighting immune factors and to stimulate development of the immune system.

The way in which this is done involves "transfer factors," tiny protein molecules which are produced by immune cells (T cells). The transfer factors are introduced to infants through the mother's milk, specifically in colostrum. The transfer factors in colostrum "transfer" immunity from the mother to the baby. Apparently, transfer factors cross mammalian species lines, meaning that when a person absorbs transfer factors from a cow's colostrum, he or she develops resistance to the pathogens to which the cow was exposed.[11]

Although the theory underlying these products isn't completely off-base, the supposed mechanism of action (again) involves immune system enhancement, which may not be a good idea. Furthermore, these transfer factors must first make it through your digestive system to be properly absorbed. However, if you believe that immune system enhancement is the answer to your problems, and digestion/absorption couldn't possibly be a problem, then by all means, put this on your list of treatment options. In my opinion, these products are overpriced because they tend to make unsubstantiated claims regarding their "secret" formulations – and manufacturers/distributors charge a premium for this "claimed superiority".

11 www.Remedyfind.com

GLYCONUTRIENTS

The study of glyconutrients is a relatively new field, and the role of glyconutrients is not completely understood. Glyconutrients are defined as foods and supplements that provide sugars along with other glycoforms (lipids and proteins) essential to the body, but which are scarce in most diets. What is known is that without glyconutrients, the body's cells are not able to communicate properly, and without proper cellular nutrition and metabolism, oxidative stress occurs. Oxidative stress results from a deficiency of antioxidants, which may be caused by inadequate diet, environmental stress, exposure to environmental toxins or any combination of these factors. Unlike popular antioxidants such as vitamins E and C, glyconutrients can supposedly eliminate free radicals inside the cells themselves and may boost production of the body's virus-killing T cells.

One company leads the field with glyconutrients. They currently have reports regarding HCV or extra-hepatic symptoms (like fibromyalgia or chronic fatigue syndrome). One doctor-initiated study of eight patients showed definite quality-of-life improvements (like greater energy and endurance). Again, on a cost/benefit basis I believe these products are over-sold and overpriced.

HOMEOPATHIC REMEDIES

The key reason I've included homeopathy here is that I have seen claims on the internet for homeopathic "cures" for Hepatitis C. I believe these to be patently false and any good homeopathic practitioner would agree.

For the sake of brevity and clarity, I've "lifted" a definition and description of homeopathy from the Encyclopedia Britannica (with attribution).

"A system of therapeutics, notably popular in the 19th century, which was founded on the stated principle that "like cures like," *similia similibus curantur,* and which prescribed for patients drugs or other treatments that would produce in healthy persons symptoms of the diseases being treated.

"This system of therapeutics based upon the "law of similars" was introduced in 1796 by the German physician Samuel Hahnemann (q.v.). He claimed that a large dose of quinine, which had been widely used for the successful treatment of malaria, produced in him effects similar to the symptoms of malaria patients. He thus concluded that all diseases were best treated by drugs that produced in healthy persons effects similar to the symptoms of those diseases. He also undertook experiments with a variety of drugs in an effort to prove this. Hahnemann believed that large doses of drugs aggravate illness and that the efficacy of medicines thus increases with dilution. Accordingly, most homeopathists believed in the action of minute doses of medicine.

"To many patients and some physicians, homeopathy was a mild, welcome alternative to bleeding, purging, polypharmacy and other heavy-handed therapies of the day. In the 21st century, however, homeopathy has been viewed with little favor, and has been criticized for focusing on the symptoms rather than on the underlying causes of disease. Homeopathy still has some adherents, and there are a number of national and international societies, including the International Homeopathic Medical League..."

Prior to the development of conventional medicines in this country, homeopathy was the number-one medicine. In Britain, the Royal family still employs homeopathic physicians, so this approach is certainly not on a level with Colloidal Silver or Essiac Tea (mentioned later). But for now, I'm listing homeopathic remedies for Hepatitis C as "dubious." As I see it, homeopathy can be used (at best) by a skilled Complementary and Alternative Medicine practitioner (like a naturopath) to help alleviate some Hepatitis C symptoms. It by no means treats or "cures" Hepatitis C.

By the way, there are plenty of responsible homeopaths who would agree that an illness as serious as Hepatitis C should not simply be treated with homeopathic medicine – just as there are many chiropractors who would never suggest that adjustments to the spine will cure everything from the flu to pneumonia. Yes, I have serious questions about the efficacy of homeopathy in general, but I'm not condemning the entire field. In the hands of a naturopathic doctor it could be a good "adjunct". Once again, I'm listing this particular therapy as "dubious" only because some practitioners and patients are claiming homeopathic remedies are effective treatments for Hepatitis C. There is simply no evidence to support that claim. Until there is, anyone who makes such claims is – in my humble opinion – a quack and a charlatan. If anything, homeopathy seems much better suited to addressing extra-hepatic symptoms of the Hepatitis C.

I know that there are additional "remedies" being touted as Hepatitis C treatments, but these are the biggest culprits with which I'm familiar. To avoid being "taken" by anyone pushing phony palliatives and suspect cures, use your common sense and follow these guidelines:

- Do your homework. Go online or to your local bookstore or library to research unknown products and therapies. Look for clinical research that's been reported in recognized medical journals that attests to the effectiveness of products or treatments you're investigating. For example, *http://www.megathistle.com* has numerous references to published and recognized scientific studies related to the active ingredient in MegaThistle.

- Consult a physician who has knowledge of natural remedies, or better yet, consult more than one knowledgeable physician about any product or regimen that you're planning to use.

- Ask, "How is this product/treatment supposed to work?" When you encounter advertising materials designed for the general public that are laced with multi-syllable Latin-derived words that you can't understand, it's probable that you aren't meant to understand. The sellers hope that by filling their ad copy with pseudo-scientific babble, you'll be impressed with their "obvious" medical knowledge. *Bull!* If you can't understand what's being said, ask your doctor or another reputable healthcare provider to "translate" for you. You can even email me, if you want.

- Remember, if it seems too good to be true, it probably is. If there truly were a major breakthrough in the treatment of Hepatitis C, it would be widely known. Don't buy into conspiracy theories claiming that the big drug manufacturers or the American Medical Association are suppressing cures to keep you dependent on high-priced pharmaceuticals. Nobody could keep that information under wraps for very long!

- Beware of anything that promises to cure a cornucopia of unrelated illnesses (this is my "athlete's foot to the plague" rule). Think: how many treatments are there that cure dozens of unrelated diseases? Yes, broad-spectrum antibiotics cure many different diseases, but all of these diseases are caused by bacteria, which are killed by antibiotics. They don't also prevent heart attacks and hangnails.

- You can also contact me and ask my opinion. See my contact information at the end of each chapter of this book.

Survivor Story:

"I was diagnosed with Hep C in the US when being treated
for something else. I could have fallen off the chair with
the shock, but my physician could tell me very little except
to stop drinking. I had a liver biopsy and it was found that
my liver was not showing any signs of cirrhosis. I decided
to go with acupuncture, Chinese herbs, and Chi Gong
(meditative Chinese exercises). I also take milk thistle daily.
So far, my levels have maintained a steady consistency (low
ALT/AST levels)? And when Western drug companies can
come up with a 100 percent cure for ALL of the genotypes
(mine is 1a, one of the hardest to cure so far!) then I will
consider taking the drugs. I just hope that happens sooner
rather than later."
            – Anita

As a fellow Hepatitis C survivor, your health and well-being are important to me. Many people have helped me, and I want to help you. If you have any questions about anything in this chapter, feel free to email me at *Ralph@HepCSurvival.com*.

New information about this disease is becoming available regularly. You can to stay up-to-date by signing up for important email notifications (and a FREE 6-part "survival" e-course) at *http://www.HepCSurvival.com*. This way, I can keep you informed with the latest news, and help you get the most out of this book. You'll also find a multitude of important resources through the website, including my analysis and commentary on new information as I discover it.

CHAPTER 6

Which Approaches Are Useless or Dangerous?

SURVIVAL SECRET

If it sounds too good to be true, or if it sounds too weird, it probably is.

The 19th century was the heyday of the patent medicine show, when wandering "snake-oil salesmen" drove their colorful wagons from town to town, selling cures to the uneducated and uninformed. Most of these medicines, which claimed to cure every conceivable ailment under the sun, contained significant amounts of alcohol, morphine or laudanum (a tincture of alcohol and opium). At best, therefore, the patients were in a pretty good mood after taking a few doses. At worst, the ingredients killed them before they succumbed to whatever diseases they had.

Today, you won't find snake oil salesman wandering the countryside – with their "shills" in tow (people hired to provide the "testimonials"). Instead, you'll find their high-tech descendents patrolling the internet, using the same techniques and tactics as their predecessors to relieve you of your money.

Beware of Snake Oil

When it comes to alternatives, I'm here to help you sort the good from the useless and the bad. As patients, we need to remember that there are many people selling "snake oil", just to make a buck from vulnerable and sometimes desperately ill people. This is reprehensible, but true. Buyer beware! I know it angers me when someone tries to take advantage of my condition by trying to sell me ineffective, unproven and possibly dangerous products with exaggerated claims. Whenever you investigate an unknown product, treatment or technology, consider the source and look for real scientific studies to back up any claims made by the purveyors and their "cheerleaders" (or shills). Use your common sense. Also, look for research published in recognized medical and scientific journals. Remember: if it seems too good to be true, it probably is.

I'm not suggesting that ALL makers and supporters of the following "therapies" are cold-blooded con artists. From my research, it's clear that some people genuinely believe in the curative powers of these technologies, potions and elixirs. What's more, I've known a number of patients who really believe they've benefited from using some of these treatments. In my humble opinion, however, these people probably benefited not from the treatments themselves, but from the "placebo effect" – the poorly understood interaction between mind and body that helps some "true believers" to apparently heal themselves. (Actually, in clinical studies it has been shown the placebo effect works about 30 percent of the time – for this reason it has to be adjusted for in true medical studies.)

That said... ladies and gentlemen, step right up and let me introduce you to the amazing, the miraculous, the magical mysteries and pseudo-scientific wonders of...

THE RIFE RAY MACHINE

Although mechanical variations and "improvements" have been made to the actual devices that employ this technology, the original machine was invented in the 1930s by a man named Royal Rife. The basics of the Rife Ray machine are fairly simple: inert gases are introduced into a vacuum tube (the "plasma tube"), and then "excited" by some form of high voltage, which is turned rapidly on and off. This rapid on/off modulation produces high-frequency sounds – or harmonics – that disrupt the cellular structure of various pathogens, including the Hepatitis C virus. These harmonics render those nasty pathogens... well, dead. From what I've read, that's about all that Rife Ray machine proponents can agree on.

To be perfectly blunt, most explanations for the efficacy of the Rife Ray machine sound like dialog from a mediocre episode of Star Trek – you know, the episodes where the writers have gotten the Enterprise crew into such an impossible situation that only sci-fi techno-babble can explain how they'll possibly extract themselves from their peril:

"Captain, if I can just reverse the polarity of the engine's dilithium crystals and combine that with a modulated tachyon beam, it might just produce a particulate wave that will disrupt the space-time continuum and free us from this blasted Klingon death web." Sure, it will.

Allegedly, Royal Rife worked out the frequency formulas for certain pathogens, so that his machine could specifically target those pathogens within an individual. Of course, there's a certain mystery about his original work – a conspiracy theory that his laboratory was destroyed by agents of the medical-industrial complex because they were threatened by this approach. Whatever...

When I first heard of the Rife Ray machine, I thought it sounded kind of cool. I'm an open minded skeptic, so I thought, "Why not?" The open mind is willing to consider things, but the skeptic wants to ask more questions. "Does it really ring true? Or does it seem like smoke and mirrors?" I didn't have to dig very deep before realizing that there was zero evidence that this machine actually works. I once spoke with a woman who had used one, and she spent a lot of money on the treatment. They aren't cheap. This woman, who was dying, couldn't say that it worked for her. She wasn't disgruntled; she just couldn't claim that it had done anything.

I classify the Rife Ray machine as blatant snake oil because there isn't a shred of evidence to support its effectiveness against HCV.

I wasn't blinded by the "science."

DR. HULDA CLARK'S "ZAPPERS"

In her book, "The Cure for All Diseases", Dr. Clark claims that most ill people have parasites that weaken their bodies, allowing disease to happen. She developed a protocol that includes an electronic device which she claims "zaps" the parasites and, in conjunction with a cleansing and detoxification diet, will solve any and all of these problems. Yeah, right.

Not surprisingly, Dr. Clark has been denounced by the FDA, and I believe her approach is right up there with the Rife Ray Machine, another fringe-dweller.

OZONE TREATMENT

The theory behind exposing the Hepatitis C virus to ozone is that this gas will alter the structure of the virus's envelope – the structure it needs to attach itself to host cells. In practice, your blood is passed through a UV machine that exposes it – and the Hepatitis C virus – to ozone before it's recycled into your body. Here's how one patient described her experience:

Survivor Story:

"During my research, I had read about ozone therapy. I went to a doctor, and he said he would be able to eradicate the virus from my system, especially since I had such a low viral load. I spoke with other people who were doing it, and they said they felt much better after treatment, but their viral loads were so high they did not think they would be cured, but they felt better. So I tried it. Not a very pleasant experience, since I have small veins and my arms were black and blue from all the needles in my arm. I did not get this virus from intravenous use, but I felt like a junkie when I was doing this treatment.

I continued with ozone for three months, and then took another blood test. At that time, my viral load doubled and my enzymes were slightly elevated. I was so upset with the doctor, and he said he was also surprised. It was then that I got the impression that I was a guinea pig for this treatment, and I was not going to continue. He stated that I probably had to get worse before I got better. I was afraid to find out.

Like I said, it is not an easy treatment. They draw blood from you and it goes into a quart size bottle and then they reinsert it into you by mixing it with the ozone stuff. On the up side, I had so much energy. I really did feel great. But, months after the ozone treatment, my blood tests were showing that my viral load was going up slowly."

– Carol

Beware of any natural remedy with no recognized (published) scientific research studies to support it.

Although there's anecdotal evidence that's both positive and negative, there's no real evidence that ozone therapy works – at least for Hepatitis C patients. The open-minded skeptic in me says, "Well, if it works, then more people will use it because it works, and you'll hear more and more anecdotal evidence about how great it is." But that's simply not the case here.

This may not be a very scientific method for appraising a treatment, but if a product or technology has genuine promise – if it's really getting results – then I would expect to hear a lot of about it. In addition, my antennae always go up whenever I hear, as I have with ozone treatments, that they cure everything from athlete's foot to cancer. One of the common themes among snake oil treatments is that they claim to treat and potentially cure just about everything that you can throw at them.

CHELATION THERAPY

Chelation therapy is a series of intravenous infusions containing disodium EDTA (EDTA is a popular acronym for the chemical compound ethylenediaminetetraacetic acid) and other substances. It is sometimes performed by swallowing EDTA or other agents in pill form. Proponents claim that EDTA chelation therapy is effective against atherosclerosis and many other serious health problems. Its use is widespread because patients have been led to believe that it's a valid alternative to established medical interventions such as coronary bypass surgery. Although EDTA has been found to be effective in removing (chelating) toxic metals and excess iron from the blood, there is no evidence that it offers any benefits to Hepatitis C patients – or, for that matter, to people suffering from a range of ailments that it can supposedly treat.

According to Dr. Saul Green, "Proponents claim that chelation therapy is effective against atherosclerosis, coronary heart disease, and peripheral vascular disease. Its supposed benefits include increased collateral blood circulation; decreased blood viscosity; improved cell membrane function; improved intracellular organelle function; decreased arterial vasospasm; decreased free-radical formation; inhibition of the aging process; reversal of atherosclerosis; decrease in angina; reversal of gangrene; improvement of skin color; and healing of diabetic ulcers. Proponents also claim that chelation is effective against arthritis; multiple sclerosis; Parkinson's disease; psoriasis; Alzheimer's disease; and problems with vision, hearing, smell, muscle coordination, and sexual potency. None of these claimed benefits has been demonstrated by well-designed clinical trials."[12]

Obviously, the Hepatitis C virus is clearly hard to kill – at least *en masse*. So, if I were to be "kind" regarding chelation therapy, I'd say that science needs to understand more clearly the mechanism by which it supposedly eradicates the virus. If I were to be brutally honest, I'd say that it's ludicrous to believe that if a particular therapy removes minerals from your blood, then it will also remove the Hepatitis C virus from your blood. That's the kind of wild leap of logic that is often made with dubious treatments and phony cures.

Chelation has been shown to remove plaque from veins and arteries, to remove metals from the bloodstream and to reduce catabolic stressors. These actions can improve host resistance and in this way can be of assistance to many patients with chronic illnesses. It is only when claimed as a treatment or cure for Hepatitis C that it becomes very suspect.

12   Green, Saul, Ph.D., "Chelation Therapy: Unproven Claims and Unsound Theories." www.quackwatch.org

COLLOIDAL SILVER

The famous essayist, H.L. Mencken, once wrote, "Nobody ever went broke underestimating the intelligence of the American public." True. But to be fair, desperate people sometimes take desperate measures, which is about the only explanation I can fathom for taking colloidal silver or any other liquid suspension of this metal.

In a report entitled "Hepatitis C and Complementary and Alternative Medicine: 2003 Update," the National Center for Complementary and Alternative Medicine had this to say about colloidal silver:

Silver is a metallic element that is found both in nature and in living organisms. Colloidal silver consists of tiny silver particles suspended in a solution. As a dietary supplement, colloidal silver is marketed with a variety of health claims, including for immunity, diabetes, cancer, and AIDS.

Silver has had past uses in medicine, dating back to the Middle Ages. However, the advent of drugs has eliminated the vast majority of these uses. Reviews in the scientific literature on colloidal silver, including by staff of the U.S. Food and Drug Administration (FDA), have concluded that:

- *The use of colloidal silver can cause serious side effects.*
- *Silver has no known role in the body.*
- *Silver is not an essential nutrient and should not be promoted as one.*
- *It has not been proven that silver has any role in immunity or any effectiveness against any diseases.*
- *The amounts of silver in silver supplements have been analyzed and found to vary greatly.*

Animal studies have shown that silver accumulates substantially in the body. In humans, this accumulation can have a serious side effect called argyria, a bluish-gray discoloration of the body, especially of the skin, nails and gums. How this happens is not fully known, but silver-protein complexes are thought to deposit in the skin and then be catalyzed by sunlight, in a process similar to traditional photography. Argyria is not treatable or reversible. Other possible problems include gastrointestinal distress, headaches and seizures.

I'll be REALLY direct here: colloidal silver bothers the heck out of me (and also the FDA). It costs very little to make, and sellers charge a premium and get rich in the process. If you ask me, it's truly despicable. But don't take my word, or that of the National Center for Complementary and Alternative Medicines (NCCAM) that this product has absolutely no place in treating Hepatitis C, or that its side effects are potentially dangerous. Enter the key words "colloidal silver" into an internet search engine, and check out the websites that appear.

One site offers page after page of information on silver products, including a guidebook containing "research studies" about colloidal silver's role in fighting antibiotic-resistant bacteria. The problem is: the author's conclusions don't actually say a darned thing about colloidal silver's bacteria-killing abilities (and what does that have to do with killing viruses anyway?) Instead, he simply insists that consumers must avoid confusion between true colloidal silver and products containing silver proteins or silver ions. In other words, "Accept no substitutions! Our phony-baloney product is much better than their phony-baloney product!"

Some proponents claim a whole breadth of uses for colloidal silver, ranging from asthma to athlete's foot. (Okay, I'm exaggerating – slightly.) They point out, for example, that silver sulphadiazine is used to treat burns. True. But A) silver sulphadiazine is not colloidal silver, B) silver sulphadiazine is applied to the skin, not ingested, and C) what does a topical burn ointment have to do with battling a virus?

Colloidal silver is the worst form of snake oil. It's heavily marketed with anecdotal evidence – often from people who have "felt better" after taking it, or who report drops in enzyme levels and viral loads. The problem with this "logic" is that liver enzyme levels are always in flux, as are viral loads. Given the continual fluctuations, the chances are that many people who start taking colloidal silver will do so as their enzyme and/or viral levels are on a downswing, making them think the "medicine" is working. Between that and the placebo effect, some people will attribute any turn for the better to whatever treatment they happen to be using at the time.

Some people are taking so many products that it's nearly impossible to attribute improvements to just one drug, as in the following example:

Survivor Story:

"In 2002, I had another biopsy, and was given a prognosis of one to three years. I was deep in the third stage [of fibrosis], and my viral load was very high. I hit rock bottom emotionally... I met a chiropractor in Lakeside, CA, who introduced me to colloidal silver. I started taking it, and immediately noticed results. Prior to that initial visit, my immune system was plummeting and I was catching everything from colds to flus, one after another. I started cleaning my house with bleach, and noticed almost immediately after starting the Silver that I did not get sick any more.
I also learned about milk thistle. I have been taking it daily from 2002. I was also diagnosed with fibromyalgia... so I started on GC-MSM and anti-inflammatory drugs. I also learned about a prescription drug called Marinol, for nausea and appetite stimulation. It's working great!"
– Iris

I would never criticize a desperately ill woman, but I have to question her reasoning here – how does she know which of these medications is "working great?" She's added too many variables. No one can convince me that ingesting silver is good for you. Yet manufacturers and retailers continue to make money hand over fist, taking advantage of the vulnerability and hopeful nature of people in a bad situation. As for you, my dear reader, if you'd like to risk becoming a human black-and-white photograph – and one who still suffers from Hepatitis C – that is your decision.

Essiac Tea

The following is an excerpt from a press release issued by the Federal Trade Commission (FTC) on April 5, 2000:

FTC Hits Internet Health Fraud in Continuation of Operation Cure All: New Cases Target Deceptive Hi-Tech Marketing Techniques

Internet health fraud continues to plague consumers looking for solutions to serious health-related illnesses. The Federal Trade Commission today announced three separate settlements with internet companies and their principal officers. The products include cetylmyristoleate (CMO) and Essiac Tea. The FTC alleges that these companies touted their products as being effective treatments or cures for various diseases, including arthritis, cancer, diabetes and AIDS, without adequate substantiation to support the claims. In addition, the FTC complaints challenge the companies' use of various types of sophisticated internet techniques, such as metatags, hyperlinks, and mouseovers, to deceive consumers about the efficacy of their products...

"The promotions for these supplements as 'miracle' cures are really reprehensible because they target people who have very serious, if not life-threatening, health conditions," said Jodie Bernstein, Director of the FTC's Bureau of Consumer Protection. "At a time when many health-conscious consumers are using the Web as a source of information, it's important to remember that claims must be truthful to meet legal standards, whether they're in the daily paper, on TV, or on the internet."

A Canadian nurse named Rene Caisse first discovered this amazing herbal formula when one of the patients in the hospital where she worked was cured of cancer. The year was 1922! The patient had received the herbal preparation from an Ojibway herbalist. She began to experiment with the four-herb formula and found it to be very effective in helping many ailments including cancer. So startling were her results that the Ontario government of Canada became involved. By 1938, Essiac came within three votes of being legalized by the Ontario government as a treatment for terminal cancer patients. Unfortunately her work was destroyed and it took years to surface again. However, the name of nurse Caisse lives on: Essiac is Caisse spelled backwards!

Michael D. Miller, d/b/a Natural Heritage Enterprises, based in Crestone, Colorado, sold Essiac Tea, as an alternative "remedy" for cancer. Essiac Tea generally is a mixture of four herbs: burdock root, sheep sorrel, rhubarb root and slippery elm bark. Miller sold the prepared tea for $14.50 for a bottle and the dried herbal mixture for $12. Miller made claims that Essiac Tea is effective in curing a number of diseases, such as cancer, diabetes, AIDS/HIV and feline leukemia. Wow, it even works for cats!

Now, contrast Mr. Miller's claims with those made by a company (on its website) that bills itself as the leading distributor of Essiac tea, the Herbal Healer Academy.

The Herbal Healer Academy states, "We do not and can not make any health claims regarding this formula, but we can supply you with the best herbs, instructions and our member testimonials. This tea is a nutritional supplement and is not recommended as the sole treatment for any ailment, especially life-threatening ones. Please consult a healthcare practitioner for personalized care. This tea has been found helpful when used in conjunction with conventional medicine protocols."

I don't have a problem with Essiac tea, per se. In fact, with the exception of colloidal silver (which is potentially harmful), I can imagine circumstances under which I'd be willing to remove every one of the oddball and folk-medicine remedies in this chapter off my "highly questionable" list.

Here are those circumstances:

- If none of these treatments made any claims for ameliorating or curing diseases unless such claims were substantiated by clinical or empirical data. The web copy above almost meets that requirement, but strongly implies that Essiac tea is an effective treatment for terminal cancer patients, despite the later disclaimer that "we do not and can not make any health claims regarding this formula."
- If nobody charged for these dubious products/services without a money-back guarantee. I almost hesitate to write this, because receiving a full refund wouldn't compensate you for the time wasted on bogus treatments – time that could have been used to pursue more beneficial therapies. But it's a start.
- If anyone caught cheating patients out of their money with bogus treatments was forced to drink enough colloidal silver to make them look like one of Matthew Brady's Civil War photos (virtually coloring them shades of silver).
- With regard to Essiac tea, in particular, where is the evidence that it does anything, and what is the supposed mechanism of action – i.e., how is it *supposed* to work?

Survivor Story:

"To date I'm not sure why I was following doctor's orders and hoping for the best. Well, the next step turned out to be the dreaded combo treatment. If there is any advice to pass on about that experience, it's run fast and run far because it's awful. At that point we went into a "wait and see if anything better comes along" therapy, where we are today. Am I doing anything different, you ask. Not really. Okay, I stopped about 95 percent of my drinking, but still play ball, workout and try to maintain a positive outlook. I did do some research on the web and found some info on supplements that might help my liver. I currently take a supplement cocktail of milk thistle, alpha lipoic acid, selenium, B complex and vitamin C. Does it help? I'm not

sure, but I'm still living pretty much the same way I was before the diagnosis. My theory is that we're all going to die anyway, so why let this bother me? Especially because I still feel pretty good. I hope this helps someone and everyone should remember that the drug companies are feverishly trying to find a cure for this bugger. Remember, if there's a buck to be made, someone out there is going to figure out how."

– Joe

COFFEE ENEMAS

Early on in my quest for ways to help my ailing liver I heard coffee enemas would help to cleanse and detoxify both the liver and gall bladder. Upon closer investigation it became clear that these claims were based on the controversial Gerson cancer therapy, of which coffee enemas are one component. The claim is that certain constituents of coffee, when taken in enema form, help the liver and gall bladder to cleanse themselves of "toxins". According to the Office of Technology Assessment, "There is no scientific evidence to support the claim that coffee enemas detoxify the blood or liver."

There is also the question of the need to detoxify the liver. Hepatitis C is a virus. While one might choose to label it a "toxin" it is not one in the true sense. So, even if coffee enemas could indeed detoxify the liver, what bearing would that have on dealing with the Hepatitis C virus? If you want to detoxify your body, the best approach is to avoid and eliminate toxins from your environment, as much as possible, and live a healthy lifestyle (as recommended in this book, and many others). This way the body can better cleanse and detoxify itself naturally.

The coffee enema is certainly one practice I would not recommend. Especially having researched it further and learned about people who went overboard with coffee enemas and actually compromised their health (including some fatalities).

KOMBUCHA TEA

This is another folk remedy that I have often heard recommended for Hepatitis C patients. In fact, it is even hailed by some as a wonder cure-all (alarm bells are ringing already).

Kombucha is a fermented drink made with sweet tea and Kombucha culture (a symbiosis of bacteria and yeast). The tea is a folk medicine known around the world under a variety of names. Here in the Western Hemisphere it is generally known as Kombucha. According to the Mayo clinic website, there isn't a single human trial that has been reported in peer reviewed literature. And, certainly not for as tenacious a virus as Hepatitis C.

Because this "tea" is often home brewed (or fermented), there are also certain dangers to be aware of. For example, aspergillus is a fungus that has been found in Kombucha tea and can be potentially dangerous; especially to people with weakened immune systems.

Other negative reactions include allergic episodes, jaundice (not a good one for someone with liver disease), nausea and vomiting, and even one suspected death (this, again, according to the Mayo Clinic website). The article mentioned closes by essentially saying that until the possible benefits and risks are better known, it is best to avoid this concoction. I agree.

As a fellow Hepatitis C survivor, your health and well-being are important to me. Many people have helped me, and I want to help you. If you have any questions about anything in this chapter, feel free to email me at *Ralph@HepCSurvival.com.* New information about this disease is becoming available regularly. You can to stay up-to-date by signing up for important email notifications (and a FREE 6-part "survival" e-course) at *http://www.HepCSurvival.com.* This way, I can keep you informed with the latest news, and help you get the most out of this book. You'll also find a multitude of important resources through the website, including my analysis and commentary on new information as I discover it.

CHAPTER 7

Is Your Food Helping or Hurting You?

Your food DOES
make a difference.

When it comes to Hepatitis C, what you *don't* do is sometimes as important as what you *do* do. In fact, you may benefit more from avoiding certain things – alcohol, the wrong types of fats and processed sugars, for example – than ingesting liver-support products and nutritional supplements. Small changes to your diet can produce big results.

I was once approached by a friend, who said, "Ralph, you're into holistic health and all that. I'd like to feel better and have more energy. What vitamins should I take?"

I replied, "Before you start thinking about vitamins, maybe you should drink less then a half-quart of Scotch a day, and stop eating only barbecued meat and canned vegetables. Eat fresh vegetables, stop eating white bread, and try more whole grains. And while you're at it, turn off the TV and get some exercise. Take brisk walks or jog on a regular basis. Start with a good multivitamin. Then, when you've done all those things, ask me which specific nutritional supplements to take."

Survivor Story:

"In addition to the herbal medicine, I continue to eat organic foods as much as possible and have taken up yoga once again after 30 years."
    – Anne

For most of us – those relatively free of hepatic and extra-hepatic symptoms, fibrosis, cirrhosis and complicating conditions – there's really no need for a crash Hepatitis C diet (they do exist, along with special Hepatitis C cookbooks, but for most survivors they are unnecessary). Instead, focus on designing and/or maintaining the kind of healthy, well-balanced diet that every human being should follow, but that so many Americans don't. FYI: by "diet," I'm referring to actual foods, not the liver support/protection products and nutritional supplements discussed in Chapters 3 and 4.

AVOID THE SAD (STANDARD AMERICAN DIET)
    Even if you weren't a Hepatitis C survivor, I would strongly urge that you avoid what's sometimes called the Standard American Diet, or SAD. It truly is a *sad* diet. You couldn't invent one that does a better job of promoting obesity and the myriad of health problems than the one that most Americans eat every day. The Standard American Diet is high in processed foods, sugar and unhealthy fats, and low in complex (plant) carbohydrates and fiber. When you eat SAD, you're on a fast track to the cemetery.

SURVIVAL SECRET

Protein is GOOD for your liver.

WHAT ABOUT PROTEIN?

There is quite a bit of misinformation about protein and the liver. Unless you are in end-stage liver disease, your body can and does readily use protein even from meat – although lean organic meat would be best, in balanced amounts, of course. This is not to say the ultra-high-protein Atkins diet would be appropriate for Hepatitis C patients.

Instead of SAD, most experts recommend the following dietary guidelines. Again, I am presenting these guidelines for Hepatitis C survivors, but nearly everyone alive could benefit by following them.

- Drink enough water.
- Don't drink alcohol.
- Avoid chemical additives and pesticides in your food.
- Eat regularly throughout the day.
- Eat a balanced diet that contains the three major food groups: carbohydrates, fats and protein.
- Eat a wide variety and quantity of fruits, vegetables and grains (preferably organic) to get phytochemicals, vitamins and minerals.
- Avoid or limit junk food, processed food, fried food, and high-sugar food.[13] Some say to limit caffeine intake. However, consider this; there have been several studies that show two or more cups of coffee per day can actually inhibit or prevent liver cancer. This may have nothing to do with the caffeine (see more on coffee later in this chapter).

13   From *Living with Hepatitis C for Dummies*, Nina L. Paul, Ph.D., Hoboken, NJ: Wiley Publishing, Inc., 2005.

BEWARE, CORN SYRUP IS EVERYWHERE!

Most of these guidelines are either common sense or common knowledge. I'm often asked, however, just why processed foods are so bad for us. To answer this question, let's focus on one of the most popular ingredients in today's processed foods – high-fructose corn syrup (HFCS). High-fructose corn syrup is six times sweeter than sugar, helps prevent frozen foods from developing freezer burn, and keeps packaged foods soft- and fresh-tasting for longer periods. In the 1970s, it began making its way into foods that used to be made with sugar or contained no sweeteners at all. (If you've ever wondered why Coca-Cola tastes different than you remember as a kid, the substitution of HFCS for cane sugar is the reason.)

Survivor Story:

"I changed my diet, which up to that point was "eat whatever I want."... I had to weed out the high amounts of sugar I was consuming and refined foods. I began to buy books on health and nutrition... I try to eat only whole foods, like raw vegetables, fruits and grains. I exercise 20 minutes a day, but mostly I have learned that you must take care of yourself like you are the most important creature in the world and understand what is good for you."
– Rita

Today, HFCS comprises nine percent of the average adult's energy intake. According to journalist Greg Critser, author of the book *Fat Land,* the body metabolizes concentrated fructose differently from sugar, more easily converting it into fat. In fact, science isn't quite certain how the body metabolizes HFCS, but it does seem to raise levels of triglycerides, which contribute to the advent of heart disease (and fatty liver disease). Also, any high-sugar diet may overload our sensitive sugar-control mechanisms, draining our systems of essential trace minerals that help maintain stable blood sugar levels, thus straining our ability to create insulin. It's probably no coincidence that the rapid spread of diabetes has occurred simultaneously with the growth of HFCS in processed foods.

Other artificial food products – including all colorings, flavorings, preservatives and pesticides – may confound or overload the body's system for digesting and detoxifying foods.

Digestion and detoxification are complex processes. Enzymes are bio-chemicals that break down food into components that are most useful to the body.

Over the generations, our bodies have developed enzymes that are aided by the antioxidants contained in various vitamins and minerals. These enzyme mechanisms have evolved as our diets have evolved – slowly. In just the last generation, however, the food industry has introduced thousands of new additives that have outstripped the ability of these enzymes to digest and detoxify.[14]

Here is another caveat regarding food. Try to limit your salt intake, because (A) too much salt is not good to begin with, and (B) it can put a strain on an otherwise compromised liver by causing fluid to build up in the body.

SURVIVAL SECRET
Avoid iron supplements.

Also, unless you have been diagnosed as anemic (iron deficient) don't supplement your diet with iron. This is one of the main reasons why people with Hepatitis C should limit their intake of red meat. In some Hepatitis C cases, too much iron can be a problem, causing a potentially dangerous condition known as hemochromatosis, so iron supplementation is best avoided by Hepatitis C survivors like us.

Of course, iron is important to your health (iron deficiency leads to anemia), but with a balanced diet you are probably getting plenty. Your healthcare provider can and should monitor your iron levels as part of your ongoing care if you've shown any signs of elevated iron levels.

14   Bissoon, Lionel, MD, *The Cellulite Cure,* Albuqurque, NM: Meso Press, 2006.

SURVIVAL SECRET

Fresh fruits and vegetables are generally better for you than canned.

PHYTOCHEMICALS

I'm also asked why fresh vegetables are better than canned. The answer is this: fresh vegetables contain much higher levels of the plant chemicals with protective or disease-preventative properties. Carotenoids, flavonoids, phytoestrogens and isothiocyanates are among the phytochemicals contained in different fresh fruits and vegetables. These act as powerful antioxidants that perform a variety of important chores – from slowing cell damage and reducing inflammation to inhibiting bone loss, lowering cholesterol and preventing cancer.

Survivor Story:

"*My diet consists mainly of high protein, good fats, and low sugar, and now I'm back at 117 lbs. I'm introducing more and more raw foods into my diet, including cleansing juices such as, pineapple/carrot/ginger. I avoid milk, soda, coffee, cigarettes and alcohol, and drink plenty of purified water and herb teas. And the "not so" palatable olive oil and grapefruit liver/gallbladder cleanse is becoming a ritual. I cheat from time to time, but I don't make it a habit. After all, it's not what you eat occasionally that is harmful, but what you eat everyday.*"
– *Debbie*

Some researchers believe that the benefits of phytochemicals are greatly diminished – if not eliminated – when fruits and vegetables are picked "green" and allowed to ripen "off the vine." In other words, they believe that the only way to ingest the needed phytochemicals is to eat fresh produce straight from the garden or the farmer's market (or in freeze-dried form). Clearly this isn't an option for many of us, but shop-bought fresh fruits and vegetables, and even uncooked, flash-frozen produce, are better than canned.

Most canned vegetables are cooked in order to help preserve them, which reduces the quantity of vitamins and minerals they contain. But don't panic. Although most of us consume more steamed, sautéed or baked vegetables than raw vegetables, and yes, this does reduce the vitamin and mineral content (which evaporates along with the steam), everything "evens out in the wash." Raw vegetables do contain more nutrients, but – even if you chew each bite the requisite 32 times – your body can't extract most of the vitamins and minerals from raw vegetables. On the other hand, while cooked vegetables contain fewer nutrients, your digestive system finds it easier to extract nutrients from foods whose fibers have been partially broken down, therefore, lightly cooked is likely best. One of the problems with canned vegetables, however, is that you're cooking them twice.

So, What Can You Eat?

Okay, I've covered the "eat less of" side of the dietary equation. On the "eat more" side, here are my personal recommendations:

- Eat more whole seeds and nuts for essential fatty acids.
- Drink more (or some) green tea.
- Get a juicer and drink my favorite combo: carrots, celery and beets with a bit of parsley.
- Eat more green foods, more raw foods, and more fresh foods.
- Fruits and veggies are your friends. Try Juice Plus+ to supplement fruits and veggies in a convenient and relatively inexpensive form. (More on this later...)
- Eat more garlic. Raw is best if you don't mind alienating your family or friends for awhile.
- Eat more cruciferous vegetables. This category includes cabbage, broccoli, and Brussels sprouts.

- Eat organic foods when possible. Your liver does not need the additional work of dealing with any pesticide residue.
- Eat whole-grain breads.
- Oatmeal with a bit of maple syrup is a much better regular breakfast than bacon and eggs – although there is little wrong with any food eaten occasionally. Brown rice cereal for breakfast is also really good.
- Switch to lean meats (especially organic) if you haven't already. They are a good source of protein. Fish and eggs are wonderful sources of lean protein.
- Drink health shakes regularly.

As also mentioned earlier, I am fortunate and grateful that I do not feel the debilitating effects that often accompany chronic Hepatitis C. This may or may not be because I've pursued natural health and wellness enhancement even before I was diagnosed. Since the diagnosis, I have simply stepped up and better focused my healthy living protocol.

You don't have to become a fanatic. Just eat more sensibly, supplement appropriately, exercise regularly, get plenty of rest and find ways to reduce stress (or to minimize its negative effects on you).

One more thing: get a "veggie wash" spray and clean your fruits and vegetables well before preparing.

Survivor Story:

"I drink a ton of water. The medicine [pegInterferon-Ribavirin] will make you quite thirsty. Try not to drink a lot of caffeine. That will dehydrate you. Especially on injection night, I would get a big 7-11 super gulp and drink that like there was no tomorrow. It made me feel a lot better all around."

– Frank

SURVIVAL SECRET

Most of us don't drink enough water.

As Frank indicates, drinking sufficient water is essential for managing some of the side effects of pegInterferon-Ribavirin therapy. For the rest of us, it just makes good sense. Why? Because the typical North American is dehydrated, a condition that – among other things – makes it more difficult for the kidneys to flush toxins from the body. In addition, it places more strain on the liver.

On average, you should drink four to eight glasses of water per day, or a total of 32 to 64 ounces. When you think about it, that's not very much water. Even 64 ounces is just four, 16-ounce bottles of water per day. And keep in mind, it is better to drink from four to eight ounces every hour than larger quantities all at once. You needn't limit yourself to water so long as you avoid drinks containing excessive sugar, especially high-fructose corn syrup. As stated on the next page, there have been studies regarding coffee and the liver that show it could be beneficial; but, even with this encouragement, I limit my intake to no more than three cups per day.

It should go without saying that alcoholic beverages are a no-no. Although I'll continue to say it, again and again.

Personally, I drink a lot of water, but I also stay hydrated with green tea. Recently I put a reverse osmosis filter under my sink to filter my drinking water. To make your water healthier and more interesting, add fresh lemon juice.

Some people are suspicious of spring water packaged in plastic containers, claiming that the plastic leaches into the water. This could be true, I suppose, but the effect would likely be negligible, in my humble opinion. However, if you can avoid it, why not do so?

DRINKING COFFEE MAY SLOW THE
PROGRESS OF HEPATITIS C

In marked contrast to the highly questionable coffee enema treatment mentioned earlier, recent studies have shown that drinking coffee daily can be beneficial to Hepatitis C sufferers.

Patients with chronic Hepatitis C and advanced liver disease who drink three or more cups of coffee per day had a 53% lower risk of liver disease progression than non-coffee drinkers, according to a new study published in the November 2009 issue of the *Journal of Hepatology.*

The study, led by Neal Freedman, Ph.D., MPH, from the National Cancer Institute (NCI), included 766 participants enrolled in the Hepatitis C Antiviral Long-Term Treatment against Cirrhosis clinical trial (HALT-C). Patients had Hepatitis C-related bridging fibrosis (a degree of disease that is close to end-stage liver disease) or cirrhosis and failed to respond to standard treatment. Each participant completed a survey of their typical frequency of coffee and tea intake.

Follow-up was conducted every 3 months during the nearly 4-year study period. Clinical outcomes were assessed, including ascites (abnormal accumulation of fluid in the abdomen), prognosis of chronic liver disease, hepatic encephalopathy (brain and nervous system damage), liver cancer, spontaneous bacterial peritonitis, variceal hemorrhage, or increase in fibrosis. Liver biopsies were also taken twice during the study.

Participants who drank 3 or more cups of coffee per day had a decreased risk of one of the clinical outcomes assessed. There was no observed association between tea intake and liver disease progression.

This is not the first study to link coffee consumption with a reduction in liver disease. Kaiser Permanente studied 125,000 people with healthy livers from 1978 to 1985 and found that the incidence of cirrhosis from alcohol consumption was reduced by 22% for each cup of coffee consumed. The findings were published in the *Archives of Internal Medicine* in June 2006.

The mechanism by which coffee protects liver function is unclear. Coffee contains over 1,000 chemical compounds. Whatever the mechanism, coffee intake is associated with the normalization of several liver enzymes that cause tissue damage and may prevent carcinogenesis.

The Hepatitis C virus is the leading cause of chronic liver disease. Globally, the World Health Organization (WHO) estimates 3 to 4 million persons contract HCV each year with 70% becoming chronic cases that can lead to cirrhosis of the liver and liver cancer.

"Given the large number of people affected by HCV it is important to identify modifiable risk factors associated with the progression of liver disease," said Dr. Freedman. "Although we cannot rule out a possible role for other factors that go along with drinking coffee, results from our study suggest that patients with high coffee intake had a lower risk of disease progression." Results from this study should not be generalized to healthier populations cautioned the authors.

SURVIVAL SECRET

Overweight people do not respond as well to Interferon treatment.

O BESITY AND THE L IVER

This fact probably indicates that being closer to your ideal weight is healthier for ALL Hepatitis C patients, even those who choose not to undergo the current therapy.

As I mentioned earlier, there are some special Hepatitis C diets and cookbooks, and there's nothing wrong with them. They espouse eating good foods, but (again) these are good foods that everyone should eat. In my view, a practical Hepatitis C diet is a healthy diet, which is dissimilar to what most Americans eat. This diet is high in natural fiber, both vegetable and grain fiber (whole grains, not processed grains), and contains complex carbohydrates, not simple sugars and/or processed sugars.

Again, some people are concerned about the amount of protein that Hepatitis C survivors should ingest. My view from conferring with medical experts is that even a sick liver can handle reasonable amounts of protein, but, as stated earlier, I wouldn't recommend the Atkins Diet. Other people advise you to avoid animal proteins, but these people tend to be vegetarians or vegans anyway.

MIDDLE-OF-THE-ROAD

As stated earlier, my approach to diet is very middle-of-the-road. On the one hand, I see no reason to go macrobiotic or embrace any other radical dietary approach. On the other, *I do not* recommend a "business as usual" approach, especially if your diet centers on Jim Beam and McDonald's hamburgers. If you eat well, you're doing more for your liver than most people. When I visit the supermarket, I often sneak peeks at what other people are putting on the conveyor belt. I've been known to say to my kids, "Look at the food they are buying – you know what? *They'd be better off eating the packaging!*" More often than not, their entire shopping carts are filled with Twinkies and Diet Coke and Puffed Wheat and Fritos and highly-processed ice cream. You look at these people, and they look like the food they eat – not very healthy. You really can see the effects of what they've been eating.

Don't get me wrong. I love the occasional sandwich with Genoa Salami and Provolone cheese, not to mention rare encounters with hot dogs topped with sauerkraut and mustard. When I first started eating more healthily, decades ago, I said to myself, "What's the point of eating healthy if I can't 'cheat' once in a while with a good hot dog?" Of course, the key word here is "occasionally." Most people, including Hepatitis C survivors, are abusing their bodies continuously, not occasionally.

When it comes to diet, please understand that I'm not referring to people with advanced liver disease. Keep in mind that, because the liver is a non-complaining organ, you may have lost as much as 85 percent of liver function before you begin noticing severe symptoms. At that point, you do have to very carefully watch your salt intake along with the amounts and types of protein you are ingesting. This is a situation that has less to do with Hepatitis C than with liver failure. This is a situation where simple dietary changes are no longer sufficient, and where medications are a necessity. This is one area where your doctor will be one of the best people to advise you on what you should and should not eat.

But until that point (which I hope will never come), a sensible and balanced diet should be enough to keep your body in tip-top condition. As I like to say, "I'm one of the healthiest people I know. I just happen to have a potentially deadly chronic disease."

Survivor Story:

"*I went through treatment and have been virus free for two and a half years. All of my liver enzyme levels are normal. I'm convinced I'm "cured". I have a couple of friends who were not successful with therapy. It could be they had a different genotype, I'm not sure. The doctors never determined which genotype I had. The only advice I can give you is don't miss any treatments, drink the gallon of water every day, eat as healthy as possible. I continued to work through treatment. It was very difficult but worth every bit of the side effects to beat this virus.*"
        – Rich

Survivor Story:

"*I lived with this for 4 more years when I met an amazing doctor who told me I was a perfect candidate for combination therapy. I was apparently the right genotype, age, sex, etc. for optimal results so i was injecting myself with this for 6 months and taking pills with it. I was very pale and sick but still worked (even though it took everything in me but it also helped to keep my mind off of my situation). It has been one year this February since taking the medication and I am still negative. I am so, so happy.*"
        – Bridgette

MY PERSONAL LIVER CLEANSE RECIPE

I'm often asked if there's a certain "liver cleanse" recipe that I use – such as olive oil, lemon and garlic – or if I employ other strategies for cleansing the liver. Here's my response: The best way to cleanse your liver is to keep harmful substances out of your body. However, the most sensible "liver flush" I've seen is recommended by Christopher Hobbs, L.Ac. By the way, cleansing once at the beginning of each of the four seasons should be often enough.

1. Take one cup of freshly squeezed orange juice. Add some lemon until the mix tastes sour. You can water down the final mix to make it more palatable.

2. Add the juice of one or two cloves of fresh garlic (using a garlic press). Grate in some raw fresh ginger root, as well.

3. Mix in one tablespoon of high-quality olive oil, blend this in (or shake it well in a glass container), and then drink it up.

4. Follow up with two cups of cleansing herbal tea. There are many available at health food stores today.

5. Drink this in the morning after a bit of stretching and deep breathing, then do not eat or drink anything else for one hour.

My recommendation is to do this for 3 to 7 days in a row during every change of season. (Incidentally, I do not like any liver flush that involves large amounts of olive oil and lemon juice. This can be a real shock and strain on your liver.)

ANOTHER IMPORTANT NOTE

No liver flush or dietary changes can compensate for frequently "splurging" on food and drink that's bad for your liver. In other words, don't assume you can scarf down a 12-pack of beer one night, and then undo any damage with a liver cleansing formula in the morning.

As a Hepatitis C patient, you have a potentially life-threatening disease. Why would you do something deliberately bad for your liver if you know it can shorten your life, or negatively impact your quality of life? There is an inherent psychological problem here that you may need professional help in addressing.

As a fellow Hepatitis C survivor, your health and well-being are important to me. Many people have helped me, and I want to help you. If you have any questions about anything in this chapter, feel free to email me at *Ralph@HepCSurvival.com.*

New information about this disease is becoming available regularly. You can to stay up-to-date by signing up for important email notifications (and a FREE 6-part "survival" e-course) at *http://www.HepCSurvival.com.* This way, I can keep you informed with the latest news, and help you get the most out of this book. You'll also find a multitude of important resources through the website, including my analysis and commentary on new information as I discover it.

CHAPTER 8

Which Nutritional Supplements Could Most Help You?

Take your vitamins!

While good sense and a proper diet will definitely go a long way towards helping you deal with Hepatitis C, you must realize that you can't possibly get all the nutrients you need from your food alone. The friend mentioned in the previous chapter who wanted to feel better and have more energy who asked me "What vitamins should I take?" was on the right track. While I thought she needed to address her food intake issues first, vitamins and other nutritional supplements are also very necessary for everyone, and especially for Hepatitis C sufferers. With factory farming and nutritionally-depleted soil, supplementation becomes increasingly important.

NUTRITIONAL SUPPLEMENTATION

At long last, medical doctors worldwide are recognizing the value of nutritional supplements. And many more doctors are now aware of milk thistle and its possible beneficial effects.

SURVIVAL SECRET
Even doctors are now recognizing the value of nutritional supplements.

According to Lark Lands, Ph.D. and Lynn Patrick, ND., there are two types of liver damage associated with chronic Hepatitis C – one caused by the infection itself; the other by the immune system's efforts to fight the virus. Even if you eat a healthy and balanced diet, you may need to supplement your diet to counteract the damage caused by these two sources.

ANTI-OXIDANTS

A process called oxidative stress plays a role in the progression of chronic Hepatitis C. Oxidative stress occurs when free radicals (unstable electrons and oxygen molecules) move through the liver causing additional inflammation and scarring. Free radicals form naturally in the body, especially when the immune system attacks an invader. The process is accelerated in chronic viral infections. The amount of damage caused by oxidative stress is linked to both the amount of liver fibrosis and the overall liver damage.

The level of the antioxidant, glutathione, is significantly depleted in many people with Hepatitis C. Insufficient amounts of glutathione can reduce the liver's ability to break down drugs, chemicals and other toxins, which can result in liver damage.

Survivor Story:

*"My good friend and I read about Hep C, and I started on
a natural supplemental daily regimen. I am still on it today.
It is my belief that the vitamins and herbs have helped me
to stay as healthy as possible. I am a strong believer in
milk thistle (especially the phytosome form), olive leaf, liver
blend and Echinacea, and I also take several others that
are blood antioxidants… The Peg/Riba treatment did not
eradicate my disease, but even today my liver function is
normal and my health is good. It will take trial and error
for each person to find their special "cocktail," but the
overall effect is worth it. Luckily, I no longer have to see
my liver specialist on a regular basis."*
      – Priscilla

Studies of people with chronic Hepatitis C found much lower
levels of the antioxidants glutathione, vitamin A, vitamin C, vitamin
E, and selenium than in people who didn't have HCV. One such
study was reported in 1996 by Dr. Barbaro and colleagues regarding
glutathione. Low levels of antioxidants are often accompanied
by high levels of blood markers that indicated damage from free
radicals. The levels of these markers could be closely correlated with
the amount of liver fibrosis. The higher the level of oxidative stress,
the more advanced the fibrosis.

The most important information such research has revealed is
that even in the early stages of Hepatitis C, antioxidants are important.
Although this information doesn't prove that antioxidants prevent
liver damage, the authors of the research suggested that antioxidants
might play an important role in slowing the progression of HCV
and delaying the onset of cirrhosis.

Nutritional antioxidants can counteract the damage caused by
oxidative stress and low glutathione levels. These include vitamins
A, E and C, the family of carotenoids (including beta-carotene)
from red and orange fruits and vegetables, the minerals zinc and
selenium, R-lipoic acid, N-acetyl cysteine (NAC), and S-Adenosyl-L
Methionine (SAMe).

In fact, the antioxidants vitamin E, R-lipoic acid, NAC, SAMe, and selenium have been studied in people with Hepatitis C to determine their effect on liver inflammation. The process of inflammation can also involve the accumulation of fat in the liver. Fatty cells are susceptible to damage, which can cause fibrosis and, ultimately, cirrhosis. Of course, the death of liver cells due to viral attack and the replacement of these cells with "scar" tissue is the most common progression of Hepatitis C to fibrosis and cirrhosis.

Vitamin E, selenium, zinc, and NAC have also been studied for their potential to inhibit fibrosis in chronic hepatitis. Of special importance are the antioxidants and nutrients that work together to increase glutathione. The use of supplements to normalize glutathione levels may be very important for preventing liver damage. The key nutrients that contribute to glutathione production are R-alpha-lipoic acid, vitamin C, vitamin E, and NAC. The B vitamins and the mineral selenium also contribute to the antioxidant defense system.[15]

SURVIVAL SECRET
Most of us do not eat enough fruits and vegetables.

FRUITS AND VEGGIES

Fruits and vegetables supply chlorophyll, enzymes and other essential micronutrients that are deficient in most modern diets. As stated earlier, organic is better. Today, in addition to eating more fresh fruits and vegetables, I also take Juice Plus+ to help make sure I am getting these essential plant enzymes and nutrients (more on that later). Another good source of information on this important subject is available at *http://www.fruitsandveggiesmatter.com*.

15   Lands, Lark, Ph.D. and Patrick, Lyn, ND. "Nutritional Supplementation." Hepatitis C Choices, Caring Ambassadors Program, 2004

Green tea is one of my beverages of choice because it contains catechins, which are said to be important immune balancers and healing substances. I drink a pot of green tea every day, unsweetened. My preferred choice is organic green tea with jasmine.

SURVIVAL SECRET

It's very difficult to get all your body's nutritional needs through just food, no matter how well you eat.

MODERN DIETS NEED SUPPLEMENTATION

Factory farms grow crops with substandard soil conditions and treat animals with hormones, antibiotics, and who-knows-what other chemicals. Many of the supplements I included on my "A-List" are good for maintaining better health in general. I also take a very good professional-grade multi-vitamin without iron.

Although MegaThistle contains phosphatidylcholine, I still supplement with additional amounts. It's been shown to be a valuable supplement for liver health. I often mix it into health shakes that I drink on a regular basis (or even just sprinkle the powdered form onto my oatmeal, for example.) Incidentally, you can find my delicious personal health-shake recipe at *http://www.HepCSurvival.com/shake*.

Survivor Story:

"I found out through the Mayo Clinic and from reading other Hep C stories that there were other alternatives. Do your research. There's not just one solution. Ask others about their stories, and once you gather your information, make your own decisions based on your life. Doctors do not have all of the answers. Doctors do not teach about alternative medicine."

– Alice

My "A-List" Group of Supplements

Since it was originally published in 2001, my "A-List" of supplements has been refined and modified. This is based on my personal experience, research, along with feedback/input from other survivors and renowned experts. I've grouped my recommendations into four specific categories to make it simpler for you to choose what's most effective, and for your convenience in recommending supplementation options for other people you care about who don't have Hepatitis C.

The reason for these lists is that there are so many substances that may be good for protecting and supporting your health and your liver, that I needed to narrow your options down to those I feel give you the most benefits for your investment. The way I look at it is that I have a potentially deadly disease, so if I need to spend a few dollars more to make sure I am taking the best supplements possible, then that's what I'll do, but I want to get the most bang for my bucks.

As already stated, there are many, many products that are good for your liver. You or I could not possibly afford to take them all. In my opinion the cost of each product chosen must be commensurate with the possible benefit(s) it delivers. More details on each supplement and brand I've recommended can be found at *http://www.HepCSurvival.com/alist*.

Essential Liver Support "A-List"

First, of course, is **MegaThistle**, the most effective form of milk thistle, the phytosome form, as detailed earlier in this book. MegaThistle is much more potent than standardized milk thistle, up to 10x more bioavailable, and clinically shown to support normal function of liver cells. The fact that it's 10x more bioavailable makes it up to 1,000% more effective than 80% standardized milk thistle... the type most commonly found in stores. A daily dose also contains 720 mg of phosphatidylcholine (more on that later). MegaThistle is also the most affordable form of this superior formula at this dosage.

Next, there's **Sho-saiko-to**, one of many herbal formulas found in the traditional Japanese medicine chest (also detailed earlier). Sho-saiko-to is produced using traditional eastern herbs that aid the liver.

The manufacturer standardizes them and produces the product using pharmaceutical-grade processes. In fact, Sho-saiko-to is considered a true medicine in Japan where it is prescribed by doctors for liver concerns, because it has been shown to protect and support liver cells. Remember, over 1.5 million prescriptions have already been dispensed in Japan for liver issues!

R-Lipoic acid (also known as Thiotic Acid) is also on my "A-List" because it has a great reputation as an antioxidant and antiviral agent, especially within the HIV community. There is a doctor in New Mexico (Burton Berkson, MD) who received quite a bit of attention with his "triple antioxidant therapy" for Hepatitis C. In his own small studies he showed it has a significant positive effect. The keystone of Dr. Berkson's therapy was alpha lipoic acid (ALA). Also included in his protocol is milk thistle extract and selenium. Since his original studies, more has been discovered about ALA and purer, more natural and more potent forms are now available, particularly R-Lipoic acid. In one instance, three patients with chronic Hepatitis C were awaiting liver transplantation. The subjects were treated with triple anti-oxidant therapy by Dr. Berkson. The constituents of this therapy were lipoic acid, milk thistle extract, and selenium. Following treatment, the patients' lab values and symptoms improved to such an extent that liver transplantation was avoided in all three subjects. The results occurred *within two weeks,* the patients' regenerated their livers fully and they were still alive and well thirty-some years later. R-Lipoic Acid is the preferred form, and 200 mg per day should be adequate, with 600 mg optimal. This is the reason the lipoic acid I recommend is of the highest quality possible.

Next is **NAC,** or **N-acetyl-cysteine.** This is readily turned into glutathione by your body. Glutathione is essential for: A) normal phase two detoxification in your liver, and for B) protecting liver cells. Both of these are very important functions. You can buy oral glutathione, but it's much more expensive than NAC, and there's also some controversy among biochemists and clinical nutritionists about whether it passes through your digestive system intact. N-acetyl-cysteine is cheaper and is known to be easily transformed into glutathione in your body. To give you an idea of its importance, consider this real-life scenario: if you are rushed to the hospital with Tylenol (acetaminophen) poisoning, the doctors will administer intravenous NAC to detoxify the acetaminophen before it destroys too many liver cells and kills you.

The final key supplement on my Essential Liver Support "A-List" is **selenium.** Use 200 micrograms per day (and it's highly recommended you don't surpass 400 micrograms). Retrospective studies in China have shown that provinces with elevated levels of hepatocellular carcinoma (liver cancer) were brought to normal levels very quickly by the introduction of selenium (200 micrograms per day, my recommended dosage) to the inhabitants' otherwise selenium-deficient diets. As someone with a liver disease, liver cancer is definitely something I want to avoid, and selenium is quite inexpensive.

LEVEL-2 LIVER SUPPORT "A-LIST"

To take your supplementation regime to an higher level of benefit, you can go beyond the essential supplements detailed above and take these additional ones, starting with **tumeric extract.** The active ingredient, **curcumin,** is reported to be especially good for liver and gall bladder inflammation. It has been getting quite a bit of good press lately. Because Hepatitis C (or any condition ending with -itis) is an inflammatory condition, supplementing with Tumeric is a no-brainer. I take half a gram to one gram per day. Please note that tumeric is not suggested for people on coumadin or with bleeding disorders because it also acts as a blood thinner. I am currently working on making a much more effective form of curcumin available to Hepatitis C patients. Look for more information about this at the website, *http://www.HepCSurvival.com.*

Then we have **Liv.52.** This supplement can be important for liver support, especially if you're exposed to toxins regularly (you can read all about Liv.52 in Chapter 3). The reason I chose it is that there is a plethora of scientific validation of its effectiveness and safety. Liv.52 has been successful with detoxifying certain substances like alcohol. For people who are in a toxic environment, or are concerned about what they ingest (such as alcohol – which is certainly not recommended), then this product may be very helpful.

S-Adenosyl-L Methionine (SAMe) has a place on my Higher-Level Liver Support "A-List" because it is considered an extremely powerful hepatoprotectant, but it is a bit more costly than many of the others. SAMe is also extremely unstable and must be purchased in blister packs. It is another valuable glutathione booster that has undergone many studies regarding liver health in Europe. The daily dosage I have seen most recommended for Hepatitis C patients is 400mg.

SURVIVAL SECRET

It's highly recommended that you buy SAMe from a reputable source in blister packs to preserve strength and freshness.

Finally we have **Phosphatidylcholine.** Phosphatidylcholine helps protect the liver against damage from alcohol, pollution, toxins, prescription and over the counter medication, mushroom poisoning, and radiation. Phosphatidylcholine (PC) is one of the most important nutrients to consume daily for optimal health. PC is found in nuts, seeds, dandelion greens, and egg yolks: foods we consume too little of to get an optimal intake of PC. For this reason, most adults do not get enough of this valuable nutrient. An inadequate intake of PC can lead to poor liver function, fatty liver, and gallstone formation. It's useful in the treatment of a wide range of liver ailments, including hepatitis, fatty liver and cirrhosis. It also helps protect the liver from damage caused by alcohol, viruses, medications, and toxins in the environment and food. In your daily dosage of MegaThistle, you're already getting 720 mg of phosphatidylcholine, otherwise it would be on my primary list on its own. I recommend an additional 420 mg because this assures you're getting over a gram each day of this very important liver protectant and cellular nutrient.

ESSENTIAL GENERAL HEALTH "A-LIST"

This "A-List" is for *everyone*, providing dietary nutritional support with benefits that go way beyond ordinary supermarket, big-box store *(e.g. WalMart, Costco)* or even health-food store vitamins. If you want the very best nutritional support available for yourself and your loved ones, follow along with me... every brand and product I recommend to you is the highest-quality professional grade.

First, take a **high-quality multi-vitamin.** Use a copper-and-iron-free formulation, because copper and iron are generally unnecessary and they are easily found in even the Standard American Diet. Also, as mentioned earlier, supplementary iron can be problematic for Hepatitis C patients.

SURVIVAL SECRET

I would still be taking many of the supplements on these lists, especially the General Health "A-List", even if I didn't have chronic Hepatitis C.

I then recommend you take a superior **vitamin C** formula, 500mg to 1000mg per day. There is some question about whether vitamin C helps to bind iron in the body, but I've seen no solid evidence that this could be a problem. In fact, some sources claim vitamin C helps to chelate (remove) excess iron from the body. Buffered C is a gentle form of vitamin C for sensitive individuals. It helps support the body's immune system, immune responses, and white blood cell function and activity. It is one of the most potent dietary antioxidants, provides nutritional support to all functions of the body, and is essential in collagen formation.

Next is an **ultra-gamma vitamin E,** 600 IU of mixed tocopherols per day, because it's a strong antioxidant and is reported to work synergistically with zinc. Incidentally, the gamma/delta form is superior in that it also assures heart health. It delivers increased levels of gamma tocopherol, the most active of the tocopherols and the form of vitamin E associated with expanded health benefits. Gamma tocopherol represents about 70% of vitamin E consumed in a typical US diet. Recent research indicates that gamma tocopherol is more effective than its alpha counterpart in reducing oxidative DNA damage and increasing overall antioxidant properties.

Finally, there's **OmegAvail**™ **Synergy TG,** a proprietary blend of high potency omega oils, featuring TruTG™ fish oil in the form found in nature.

This ensures unmatched triglyceride (TG) potency – only fish oil blends and concentrates containing the TruTG™ seal are 90+% triglyceride bound omega-3 fish oils. Did you know that all other products claiming triglyceride bound omega fats are no more than 60% TG? As found in nature – eicosapentaenoic acid (EPA) and docosahexaenoic acid (DHA) are found naturally in fish in the triglyceride form. Research shows enhanced bioavailability of triglyceride bound omega fats over ethyl ester forms.

This unique formula contains a blend of wild deep-sea sourced fish oils containing the omega-3 fats (EPA/DHA) in the TruTG™ form, the omega-3 fat alpha linolenic acid (ALA) from flax seed oil and the most important omega-6 fat, gamma linolenic acid (GLA), from borage oil. EPA helps keep GLA metabolism in an anti-inflammatory mode. In addition, docosahexaenoic acid (DHA) plays as many important roles in human health as EPA, with an added benefit to brain function.

OmegAvail™ Synergy TG delivers these four beneficial fatty acids in one softgel: EPA and DHA from fish oil, GLA from borage oil, and ALA from flax seed oil. It includes TruTG™ fish oil which contains a minimum 90% natural TG bound omega 3 oil. These DFH fish oils are molecularly distilled to ensure purity and the removal of heavy metals, pesticides, solvents, PCB's, and other contaminants.

Fatty acids are essential to good health, and this product assures you are getting the best quality of the best fatty acids, in the best proportion/ratio.

LEVEL-2 GENERAL HEALTH "A-LIST"

For the highest level of support for everyone, add the following supplements to your daily regime.

First, use a quality **digestion aid** such as **Digestzymes**. I use this myself and recommend it because most people don't chew well enough, and digestion begins in the mouth. If your food is not digested properly, your body will not be able to absorb the nutrients your food contains. The pancreas produces enzymes that are required for digestion and absorption of food. Enzymes secreted by the pancreas include lipases that digest fats, proteases that digest proteins, and amylases that digest starch.

The health of the digestive tract is crucial for overall health of the body. If you cannot digest your food and eliminate toxins well, you don't stand a good chance of being optimally healthy, whether or not you have liver disease. In addition, virtually every chronic condition will get worse if the intestinal tract accumulates toxic by-products. Production of our own digestive enzymes declines 1% every three years after age thirty. It's understandable why so many patients need to supplement your body's naturally-produced enzymes for optimal digestion and assimilation of nutrients from food. Symptoms of deficiency of digestive enzymes include gas, bloating, constipation, malabsorption and a feeling of fullness after eating only a small quantity of food.

The proteases are important in preventing tissue damage during inflammation, and in the formation of fibrin clots. Fibrin promotes inflammation by forming a wall around the area of inflammation that results in the blockage of blood, and leads to swelling. Fibrin can also cause the development of blood clots that may dislodge and produce strokes or heart attacks. Pancreatic enzymes are useful in the treatment of many acute and chronic inflammatory conditions.

Survivor Story:

"I find that I do well when I am disciplined about taking my supplements. If I slack off, I feel run down and my joints ache. I am very thankful that I have been able to live a very active life over these past ten years. I am positive

*that my relationship with God has been the largest part
of my personal coaching in learning to live with the disease.
I have learned some of life's greatest lessons because I have
HepC. I have learned to be thankful I am alive. I can still
help others find peace."*
– Nelson

I then add **zinc** supplementation. Zinc levels have been shown to be below average in individuals with chronic liver disease. Zinc deficiency is known to suppress the immune system, but most experts believe that taking at least 30 mg per day will compensate for the deficiency.

Zinc is a very strong anti-viral element. As you may know, warts are caused by a virus. When my son Michael was 8 years old, he had plantar warts on his feet, and went through different treatments, cutting, freezing, and burning them off. This was very painful and unpleasant, to the point where Michael would refuse to go back to the doctor. So we consulted with an expert in nutritional medicine, who recommended zinc therapy. Within six weeks, the warts fell off, never to return!

The liquid **Vitamin D-3** I recommend provides *cholecalciferol,* a highly bioavailable form of vitamin D, in a nutritious, olive oil base. Vitamin D has been the subject of intensive research which has greatly increased our understanding of vitamin D deficiency. This research has also expanded the range of therapeutic applications available for cholecalciferol. Physiologic requirements for vitamin D may be as high as 4000 IU per day.

Vitamin D really isn't a vitamin at all – it was misclassified early on. It is actually a potent neuroregulatory steroidal hormone. It has become very clear that vitamin D deficiency is a growing epidemic across the world and is contributing to many chronic debilitating diseases. In the United States, the late winter average vitamin D is only about 15-18 ng/ml, which is considered a very serious deficiency state. Meanwhile, it's thought that over 95 percent of U.S. senior citizens may be deficient, along with 85 percent of the American public.

In a paper published in the August 2009 issue of the American Journal of Clinical Nutrition, Anthony Norman, an international expert on vitamin D, identifies vitamin D's potential for contributions to good health in the adaptive and innate immune systems, the secretion and regulation of insulin by the pancreas, the heart and blood pressure regulation, muscle strength and brain activity.

Access to adequate amounts of vitamin D is also believed to be beneficial towards reducing the risk of cancer.

Norman also lists 36 organ tissues in the body whose cells respond biologically to vitamin D, including bone marrow, breast, colon, intestine, kidney, lung, prostate, retina, skin, stomach and uterine tissues. According to Norman, deficiency of vitamin D can impact all 36 organs. Already, vitamin D deficiency is associated with muscle strength decrease, high risk for falls, and increased risk for colorectal, prostate and breast and other major cancers.

An unrelated study also suggests that low vitamin D is associated with Parkinson's disease. The majority (55 percent) of Parkinson's disease patients in the study had insufficient levels of vitamin D.

Meanwhile, the American Academy of Pediatrics has doubled its recommendation for a daily dose of vitamin D in children, in the hopes of preventing rickets and promoting other health benefits. The new guidelines now call for children to receive 400 international units (IU) of vitamin D per day, beginning in the first few days of life. "…Evidence has shown this could have life-long health benefits," said Dr. Frank Greer of the American Academy of Pediatrics. In a very recent study, vitamin D supplementation has also been found to increase the effectiveness of medical treatment for Hepatitis C.

SURVIVAL SECRET

Vitamins alone can't replicate the nutrients found in fresh fruits and vegetables.

Finally, use a good-quality **fruit-and-vegetable** supplement such as **Juice Plus+,** the next best thing to fresh fruits & vegetables.

As mentioned earlier, the standard American diet stinks. Even when you know this and want to eat better, good nutrition takes time and planning. Clinically proven Juice Plus+® helps you bridge the gap between the 7–13 servings of fruits and vegetables recommended by The United States Department of Agriculture (USDA) and the nutrition you actually get with your busy schedule.

Putting the right foods into our bodies is a daily struggle. Fast food drive-thrus and all-you-can-eat buffets lurk on every corner. Fat, salt, and sugar have been added to almost every package on the shelf at the grocery store. Grabbing a bag of chips or a can of soda at the convenience store is certainly a lot easier than peeling an orange or tossing a salad.

You've heard it all your life: "Eat more fruits and vegetables." Now, medical science is telling you, too. But knowing is easy. It's doing it that's hard. People turn to vitamins and other nutritional supplements to improve their diets. But vitamins alone can't begin to replicate the thousands of different nutrients found in fresh fruits and vegetables. The latest clinical research shows that people can improve their chances of living longer, healthier lives by eating more fruits and vegetables. This research is leading more and more doctors and other health professionals to recommend Juice Plus+.

You see, Americans don't simply suffer from a vitamin deficiency; we suffer from a whole-food deficiency. Juice Plus+ is not a vitamin supplement, providing a narrow range of handpicked nutrients, it's a whole-food-based product providing the wide array of nutrients found in a variety of 17 different fruits, vegetables, and grains. Each ingredient is specially selected to provide a broad range of nutritional benefits. Juice Plus+ is a complement to a healthy diet, a simple, convenient, and inexpensive way to add more nutrition from fruits and vegetables to your diet, every day (in capsule form).

You can learn about all the benefits of Juice Plus+ by going to *http://www.HepCSurvival.com/jp.*

BLUEBERRIES ARE ESPECIALLY POWERFUL

In a scientific study published in August 2009, a chemical found in blueberry leaves has shown a strong effect in blocking the replication of the Hepatitis C virus, opening up a new avenue for treating chronic HCV infections. Looking for a natural nutritional treatment for Hepatitis C, Hiroaki Kataoka and colleagues at the University of Miyazaki uncovered a strong candidate in the leaves of rabbit-eye blueberry (native to the southeastern U.S.).

They purified the compound and identified it as blueberry leaf proanthocyandin (a polyphenol similar to the beneficial chemicals found in grapes and wine). While proanthocyandin can be harmful, Kataoka and colleagues noted its effective concentration against HCV was 100 times less than the toxic threshold, and similar chemicals are found in many edible plants, suggesting it should be safe as a dietary supplement.

Using a test called ORAC (Oxygen Radical Absorbance Capacity), researchers have shown that a serving of fresh blueberries provides more antioxidant activity than many other fresh fruits and vegetables.

In a U.S. Department of Agriculture (USDA) laboratory at Tuft's University in Boston, Massachusetts, researchers have found that blueberries rank #1 in antioxidant activity when compared to 40 common fresh fruits and vegetables. Concord grape juice is next on the list with about two thirds of the antioxidant activity of blueberries followed by strawberries, kale, and spinach.

I have known about the powerful antioxidant properties of blueberries for some time. I buy Wyman's frozen wild blueberries (research has also shown that wild blueberries are much higher in antioxidant activity than cultivated ones). I use them on my granola, in shakes, smoothies, etc. and probably consume one to two 15 oz. bags per week.

Beware of anyone offering any blueberry extract with 45% proanthocyandin. First, it is likely fruit-based, not from the leaves of rabbit-eye blueberry (as the study used) and second, the proanthocyandin may be derived from other sources and added to the formula. This would not at all have the same effect as found in the study. Don't be misled – be sure it's from rabbit-eye blueberry leaves.

QUALITY CONTROL VARIES WIDELY

With regard to supplements, your best bet is to choose brands that can only be acquired through licensed health professionals, as they represent greater value overall due to their higher absorption or potency. At the very least, go to your local health food store rather than some chain store that just happens to carry vitamins. Better yet, get them from a professional source. As a licensed healthcare provider I will help you with this when you go to my website, *http:// www.HepCSurvival.com.*

SURVIVAL SECRET

Not all standard supplements (like vitamin C, etc.) are created equal.

WHERE TO GET YOUR SUPPLEMENTS AND WHY

Why should you buy your supplements through a licensed or certified health care professional instead of the health food store or elsewhere?

Let's face it, most people expect all nutritional supplements, such as vitamins, minerals and herbs to be exactly the same from company to company. With this false assumption in mind, it makes perfect sense to buy the cheapest possible products. Unfortunately, uniformity of effectiveness is *not* the case. Supplement quality can vary tremendously from company to company. This can not only determine how well a supplement works, but whether it creates side effects ranging from minor annoyances to major inconveniences.

Survivor Story:

"I have read about various vitamins and herbs that are supposed to be helpful. Through trial and error I have wound up on my own treatment which, in my case, involves living with the virus in a healthful coexistence. I think with any chronic condition a person has to become their own advocate and learn all they can, then decide for

themselves what course they want to take. I feel that if I continue to take care of myself I can maintain an active, normal lifestyle and not die from liver failure even though the virus continues to reside in me. I currently take quite a few vitamins and supplements every day, both for my liver and for my general health."
— *Richard*

So how can quality best be determined in a supplement? In answering this question, it's important to remember that nutritional supplements are processed foods, just like the bag of potato chips or can of beans that you might buy in a supermarket. In the case of supplements or herbs, the nutrients or phytochemicals have usually been packaged for purchase several days, weeks, or months after manufacture. What concerns would you have when purchasing a bag of potato chips or a can of beans? Most likely, they would be these:

1. *How fresh is the product?* No matter how carefully a processed food is packaged, eventually oxygen and age will take their toll, causing food to oxidize or, in simpler terms, rot. Therefore, most people would like to get processed food that has only spent a short amount of time on the shelf or in a warehouse.

2. *Can my body use the nutrients?* Has the food been processed to the point where the body regards it as a foreign substance and can no longer absorb the nutrients it contains.

3. *Do the contents match what is on the label?* Has the processing company, knowingly or unknowingly, added substances to the product that are not indicated on the label, or are indicated in the wrong amount? Or even worse, are the food substances on the label not even the product? No government body or private organization polices this, though *http://www.consumerlab.com/* has identified a real problem with non-professional supplements.

4. *Has the product been analyzed for microbial contamination?* Given past concerns about contamination with E.coli, melamine, heavy metal, and others, this point is particularly important. What kind of analysis has been done, and how extensive?

5. *If there is a problem, can I talk to a representative from the manufacturers?* If problems arise, we all want to talk to someone "in the know" who can resolve issues. This is essential since it is very difficult for the consumer to determine any of the above points before the food is ingested. It is also nice to know that a trusted, highly reliable person stands behind the product.

How do the above points relate to nutritional supplements? Let's examine them one at a time:

1. *Freshness.* Most nutrients (especially B and C vitamins) and herbs oxidize very readily over time, no matter how carefully they are processed and packaged. Therefore, it is important that nutrient and herbal manufacturers buy small lots that are quickly processed and made available to the consumer as soon as possible. Unfortunately, because it is more cost effective to buy large lots that are stored in warehouses for several months at a time, this is what most mass market manufactures do. Because the smaller, higher-quality companies with which we deal make freshness a top priority, it costs a little more to make the product and, therefore, these companies must charge more to stay in business. However, you get the reassurance of knowing that you are actually getting your money's worth.

2. *Nutrient availability.* Because it is more cost effective, many nutrient or herbal companies highly compress the constituents into small, very hard tablets or cram them tightly into capsules. Moreover, because the companies very often lack the equipment, they do not check and see how readily these tablets or capsules break down in the digestive tract. As a result, the saying, "Americans have the world's healthiest toilets," is more often than not true. The companies with which we deal manufacture their supplements with digestibility in mind, which is constantly verified by scientific testing. Of course, this also adds a marginal amount to the cost of the product. But there again, it also adds multiples to the value of the product.

3. *Contents of the supplements.* Because the nutrient and herbal industries are poorly regulated from a manufacturing standpoint,

far too many instances exist where an unknown substance is added, something important was never included, or a combination of the two occurs. The companies supplying our products provide 100 percent assurance that what is on the label is exactly what is in the bottle. They back up this claim with scientific testing of each batch. Again, this adds a little to the cost of the production.

4. *Microbial and toxic contamination.* The companies with which we deal analyze both the raw materials and the finished products for microbial and toxic contamination. What is that reassurance worth to you with an impaired liver?

5. *Reaching a manufacturer's representative.* Sadly, it is a known fact that many supplements available in the health food stores are manufactured by different companies at different times, depending on which company offers the lowest price. Therefore, even though the labels may look the same, the quality of the product may vary greatly from batch to batch. While this manufacturing method ensures the cheapest price, it makes it very difficult to track down the manufacturers for any particular batch. Furthermore, as you might expect, manufacturers know this and may relax their standards on the above-mentioned points. The companies we deal with maintain a staff of highly-trained professionals who can quickly and expertly answer any concerns that may arise. As you might expect, this also adds to the cost of the product. But clearly, if you truly care that the supplements you ingest can actually help, the incremental price increase is well worth it.

In light of these facts, ask yourself this question: is it better to spend a little less on products that give questionable, unpredictable results, or a little more on those that are backed by reliable, trustworthy professionals and provide much more consistent, satisfying results? If your answer is the latter, you have come to the right place. Be sure to visit *http://www.HepCSurvival.com* for all the details on getting the best professional-quality supplements for yourself.

POSSIBLE INTERMITTENT ADDITIONS

There are other supplements that I take on an intermittent basis that may be recommended by more "natural-oriented" healthcare providers. These supplements include, but are not limited to:

- Schisandra (used in China for liver ailments)
- Dandelion root (a great diuretic and mild liver cleanser, but people tend to make too big a deal about it regarding Hepatitis C)
- Coenzyme Q10 (shown to have immune boosting properties)
- Licorice root (used intravenously in Japan and other countries for hepatitis treatment, used orally by me – be cautious with this one if you have high blood pressure as it tends to raise blood pressure at higher doses.) It is already in Sho-saiko-to.
- Astragalus (considered a general tonic to the immune system)
- Pichoriza (said to be similar in action to milk thistle)
- Maitake, shitake and other medicinal mushrooms (generally antiviral and immune system balancers)
- Organic liver extract (to help provide essential nutrients)
- Eclipta Alba (widely considered a powerful liver tonic and rejuvenator).

NARROWING YOUR CHOICES

There are many other potentially helpful substances, but I've listed the ones above because their use is supported by clinical evidence or a strong biochemical rationale. Some websites are hawking dozens of supplements specifically for people with Hepatitis C. One site positions itself as providing products taken by the site owner to "cure" Hepatitis C. He's written a book claiming to have "cured" himself naturally.

If you were to take everything he offers to treat Hepatitis C on that website, you'd go broke. If this is really what he used to get rid of the virus, this person must have been rich just to be able to afford all that stuff (and "if" is the operative word here). Remember, 15 percent of people clear the virus naturally, and this guy shows no before-and-after blood tests on his website. And, if after many, many years online he still doesn't have even one testimonial of a "cure" from someone else who's followed his recommendations, it kinda makes me wonder. How about you?

I'm not saying everything being sold on this particular "cure" site is ineffectual or worthless. Many are beneficial supplements, but have little real value regarding Hepatitis C. Actually, I think he and his site mostly push frozen thymus extract because he makes the most money with it, and has all but cornered the market on that particular product.

Many other good supplements are also being given too much credit for being able to make a difference for Hepatitis C survivors. These include, but are not limited to, cats claw, burdock root, aloe vera, olive leaf, NADH, alfalfa, bee pollen, magnesium, vitamin K, barley grass powder, and Acetyl-L-Carnitine.

Survivor Story:

"I found out I had Hepatitis C nine months ago. I probably have had it longer and wasn't really aware. I am dealing much better with it now. At first, I was devastated. I was so sad I could not eat and stayed in bed all day. I prayed a lot and cried a lot. I refuse to take the treatment because it is no promise of a cure. So, I try to stay as healthy as possible mentally and physically. I continue to pray that one day soon they will find a bona fide cure. I do have scarring on my liver, but also pray about that so I can at least have some peace about it. I am lucky I have health insurance. I am sixty years old so I opt not to take the treatment also because of the side effects I've heard so much about. I just take milk thistle for now."

– Lonny

A NOTE OF CAUTION

Avoid very high doses of vitamins A and D. Over 5,000 i.u. of vitamin A can be dangerous unless monitored by your doctor, as well as more than 4,000 units of vitamin D in its cholecalciferol (best) form.

I am always on the lookout for new, credible remedies or liver support products. To stay updated, simply sign up for the updates at *http://www.HepCSurvival.com*. That way, you can stay informed about any new and relevant information, and benefit from all the ongoing legwork and research I conduct for myself and others like you and me with Hepatitis C.

As a fellow Hepatitis C survivor, your health and well-being are important to me. Many people have helped me, and I want to help you. If you have any questions about anything in this chapter, feel free to email me at *Ralph@HepCSurvival.com*.

New information about this disease is becoming available regularly. You can to stay up-to-date by signing up for important email notifications (and a FREE 6-part "survival" e-course) at *http://www.HepCSurvival.com*. This way, I can keep you informed with the latest news, and help you get the most out of this book. You'll also find a multitude of important resources through the website, including my analysis and commentary on new information as I discover it.

CHAPTER 9

Are Your Lifestyle Choices Supporting You?

SURVIVAL SECRET
Change can be good.

I
If you were to believe everything you read in the media, you'd think that we North Americans live in a society of idiotic extremes. You're either a gun-totin' bible-thumpin' conservative or a secular anything-goes liberal. You're either a beer-guzzling chip-chewing couch potato or someone who bungee-jumps off the Hoover Dam in the morning before hang-gliding over Death Valley in the afternoon. You either eat Triple-Whoppers for breakfast, or vegan hors d'oevres as your dinner's main course.

Survivor Story:

"Two years ago, I never thought I would be around this long. But thanks to a lot of lifestyle changing, a couple of good doctors, and a little more positive attitude, I'm still here."
  – Jess

These are the perceptions that discourage Hepatitis C survivors from making needed lifestyle changes – changes that are moderate, incremental and incredibly beneficial. Call me an extreme moderate, but I believe it's more important to actually perform ANY exercise – and stick with it – than to formulate some grandiose plan for dropping 50 pounds in five weeks, only to quit after realizing this was a completely unrealistic goal.

When it comes to exercise, start off easy and work your way up. When it comes to stress reduction: choose whichever methods work best for you, as long as they don't include alcohol or other dangerous chemicals (and, preferably, no chemicals at all).

EXERCISE

Some benefits of exercise:
  – Boosts energy levels
  – Improves immune function
  – Helps weight control
  – Improves sleep patterns
  – Increases muscle and bone strength
  – Relieves stress and anxiety

Regular exercise improves so many metabolic functions that it can't help but support an impaired liver (depending, of course, on the degree of impairment). In general, exercise improves your digestion and the movement of your bowels. It massages your internal organs (including your intestines) and keeps things moving through smoothly – provided you also stay well hydrated. Regular exercise also helps your blood flow more efficiently, and encourages deeper respiration, which provides more oxygen to the entire body.

(Obviously more oxygen is a good thing – consider this, how long can you hold your breath?)

Survivor Story:

"During therapy, the one thing that kept me going was to keep going. At the treatment center I saw an interesting thing. The people who worked at physically demanding jobs were responding better than the sedentary ones. The more I worked out and did cardio type activities, the better I felt. Another person in my office was diagnosed about the same time as I was. He stayed home in bed. I continued to work 8-10 hour days. He got sicker. I got better. It took a lot of determination to go out and face every day with the pain, but the more that I did it, the easier it was. KEEP GOING!"
    – Daniel

If you're exercising strenuously enough, you'll be sweating, which also aids detoxification – not that you need to overdo it. It's sometimes said that your skin is your "third kidney," meaning perspiration helps remove toxins, so there's less strain on the liver. This is one reason why many people feel elated – sometimes euphoric – after exercising. The other reason is the endorphins, or natural morphine-like substances, that are secreted during strenuous exercise. Again, you needn't go to extremes with your exercise regimen. One half-mile walk per week is probably too little exercise, but bench pressing 400 pounds (with 30 repetitions) every day is probably a bit extreme.

WALKING MAY BE YOUR "BEST" EXERCISE

As for walking, start with short distances, but do it regularly. You'll find you want to walk more often and a little bit farther over time. I was a runner for 14 years and my goal was always to run at least four days a week. Okay, that may not be necessary for you. On the other hand, if you're the kind of person who double-parks in front of the supermarket to avoid walking an extra 10 feet, I'm going to draw the line here. Some exercise is better then nothing, but it's not much better. To get started, try walking at least a mile every other day (three- to four- times a week). If you drop below three days a week, you're losing any training effects, and it's like starting over from scratch each time you walk again.

You really need the consistency of effort because otherwise you're always starting over. Look around and you'll notice that most people don't walk enough; they don't use their bodies. It's true that getting some exercise is better than what most people do, so I'm suggesting you strive for the "optimum minimum" when it comes to exercise. In my opinion, the optimum minimum is a mile every other day, at an average walking speed of 20 minutes per mile, or three miles per hour.

Walking is part of a good exercise regimen, but it's not enough. Progressive resistance exercise is also important. I've never been a big gym person (although I was once a fitness consultant and trainer at a health club), but I believe exercises such as push-ups, sit-ups, squat thrusts, jumping jacks, chin-ups, dips and pull-ups are important. Obviously, you don't need to join a gym, or even purchase weights, to perform these particular exercises. Personally, I like to alternate between different types of exercises to avoid getting bored. Although I was an avid runner, I wouldn't only run. I would also ride a bike, swim, and I even taught myself how to skip rope. Keep things interesting by choosing a variety of ways to stay physically active. It's very important for someone who has an impaired liver to stay as active as possible. Anything that keeps your body toned and fit is a good bet.

There are so many different programs that people can choose from today that there's no excuse for not becoming more active. In general, people just don't get enough exercise... period. I know one guy who traded in his riding mower for a push mower in order to get more exercise. Over just one summer, he claims to have lost 15 pounds from cutting his half-acre lawn. In addition, he believes it's very peaceful to be out in the yard, alone with his thoughts, which brings us to the subject of stress relief...

Survivor Story:

"I used to drink beer but gave up drinking over 10 years ago. I watch what I eat. I try to keep my weight around 175 pounds and I am 5'9" tall. I joined a gym which I go to three times a week. I stay away from fats and grease and most meats. I also stay away from sugars as much as possible. The only thing I take beyond everything else is the phytosome form of milk thistle. I firmly believe that milk thistle is keeping my enzyme levels down. I have taken three capsules a day (of the phytosome form) for the last five years or so and every time I have blood work done (every three months or so) my enzyme levels remain low. My gastro recommended therapy but I did research on it and felt it is too risky for me. The side effects would be too much for me to bear. Plus, there is no guarantee of improvement. If some day my condition gets worse, then I'll reconsider therapy, but not now. All I can say is to live clean and healthy, stay away from booze altogether, don't smoke, watch what you eat, join a gym and keep a positive attitude."
– Anthony

SURVIVAL SECRET

Stress inhibits healing.

STRESS RELIEF

Yoga, T'ai Chi and Qigong, as well as meditation, breathing exercises and prayer are among the methods frequently recommended to Hepatitis C patients to reduce stress. Various types of therapeutic massage, acupuncture and acupressure are also cited. But again, whatever works best for you is what you should use. I know one guy who swears by Bob Ross – the 30-minute oil painter with the red-haired "Afro" whose show still re-runs on many PBS stations. Whenever my friend is feeling anxious or aggravated, he plays one of his recorded Bob Ross episodes, and within minutes, the host's gentle and soothing voice calms him into a near trance – to the point where he often falls asleep. Do whatever works best for you.

Survivor Story:

"I am learning that STRESS takes a huge toll on our bodies, and that this is KEY in taking care of our illness. If we cannot get our stress and emotions under control, all of the healthy things we do for ourselves will amount to nothing."
     – Rita

Currently, I perform only one yoga exercise regularly, and that's the Sun Salute (Surya Namaskar). It's a multi-part exercise that I try to do every morning. It's relatively easy for anyone to learn and do. You can see a demo at *http://www.HepCSurvival.com/yoga*. I like it because it does so many things: it stretches most of your joints, and you breathe in concert with the movements, so it helps with your respiration. In addition, it massages your lymphatic system and stretches your spinal cord. I always look for things that offer the greatest benefit for the least effort/cost, and this exercise is one that anybody can learn. The more repetitions you do, the better. I try to repeat at least six times, one after the other. It's a great way to wake your body in the morning.

T'ai Chi is a moving meditation that centers your mind on your breath and your movements. Because that's so different than what most of us do during the day and in our daily lives, it really does reduce stress, much like any other form of meditation. But instead of focusing on a certain chant or a mantra, you focus on the movement, and it's that focus of attention that has a therapeutic effect, a relaxing effect. A newly-popular variant of T'ai Chi is Qigong – or Chi Gung. You can buy DVD instruction for either one online.

Survivor Story:

"This is probably the silliest sounding thing, but it really works. SMILE. Smile A LOT. It changes the attitude of the people around you, as well as yourself. I don't know why it works, but I know I would rather be around people who smile than people who looked like they just swallowed dirt. So I have learned to smile."
     – Betty

Some people enjoy meditating using guided imagery audio. Any of them are worth trying if you actually do them. I'm not referring to movement video, just the ones you throw into your CD or mp3 player, and listen to as they guide you through your breathing and your focus. Those are all worthwhile, as long as you enjoy them.

Breathing exercises are probably the easiest and most effective stress reduction techniques. There are many books written on the subject. Much of yoga science and certain meditative techniques are based on breath control or pranamaya (its Sanskrit name). *The Science of Breath* by Swami Rama is one of my favorites. A newer title is *The Art of Breathing* by Nancy Zi, which can be quite helpful, too. The advantage of using breath strategies and techniques is that they can be employed anywhere, any time.

Chanting and toning can also calm the mind and body, and there are plenty of books and CDs available on these subjects, as well.

Survivor Story:

"I don't know how long I've had Hepatitis C. I was diagnosed about a year ago. No treatment yet. I'm kind of scared but mostly grateful and appreciate another day a little more and try to enjoy life a little more."
– Ike

For some people, knitting a scarf is the best form of relaxation. Others find peace in fishing, and still others like to take a walk through the woods.

Do what you love.

Do what brings you joy.

At minimum, turn off the TV and the radio once in a while. Shut down all of the sensory bombardment that accompanies life in the 21st century, and take time to do something more 19th century.

Get out of the city if you live in one, and take a walk along the beach. Paint, if that's what you like to do. If you live in a suburban or rural area, try your hand at gardening. Go ahead and get your hands dirty. Cut your grass with a push mower.

A short list of things to do to help yourself feel better (with some repetition from above):

- Listen to music
- Be creative (art, cooking, etc.)
- Be around and play with pets and domestic animals.
- Find humor, comedy and laughter wherever you can
- Spend quality time with family, friend and loved ones whenever possible
- Get out into nature regularly
- Meditate
- Pray
- Exercise

Finally, I would be remiss if I didn't recommend massage therapy for stress reduction. Even one full-body massage per month could make a big difference in your ability to deal with the stress of daily life.

As you've likely noticed by now, most of my recommendations for Hepatitis C patients aren't very different from recommendations I might make for anyone who wants to be healthier, live better and live longer. The only reasons I make them here is that so few people are actively taking steps to be healthier, live better and live longer. Plus, so few books on Hepatitis C properly address these aspects.

Survivor Story:

"For several years I felt something was wrong in my body. I was living a healthy lifestyle and had no reason to be as tired as I was all the time. After visiting three different doctors with my complaints one of them finally tested me for Hep C. I was completely in shock at the positive result. Although I knew I had risk factors, I never in a million years thought I could have actually have it. I cried myself to sleep that night and was pretty much devastated for the next several weeks. When I finally pulled myself together I got on the internet and started to learn all I could about the virus. At first, most of the information scared the heck

out of me. But, the deeper I dug and the more I learned, the less afraid I became. Yes, it is a very serious condition and it may be what I eventually die from, but the odds are it won't be. At least 75 to 80 percent of those diagnosed with Hep C will never be really sick from it. Particularly if you take care of your emotional and physical health. My genotype is 1a and the liver biopsy I had five years ago indicated stage 1, grade 1. Because of my genotype and the fact my liver is in good shape I choose not to do the current medical therapy. My doctor agreed that this was a wise choice for now. If I start showing signs of liver disease, maybe I'll reconsider the therapy. But, for now, I am living the healthiest lifestyle I can. I don't drink alcohol or smoke cigarettes. I make sure that I eat right, exercise regularly and get plenty of rest. At first I was taking all kinds of herbs and vitamins but have narrowed it down to those I feel are most important. I take a high quality multi vitamin without iron, extra vitamin C and E, along with CoQ10 and alpha lipoic acid. One of the most important herbs I take is (ed: the active ingredient in MegaThistle)."
    – Debbie

SURVIVAL SECRET

Alcohol may be the sick liver's worst enemy.

ALCOHOL

In my opinion, ongoing alcohol use is the number-one cause of death among Hepatitis C patients.

Let's face it: many people contracted Hepatitis C from intravenous drug use, and even if they're no longer using drugs, they still may not have the best coping skills. So, what's the most socially acceptable way to cope? Alcohol. That's probably what exacerbates most people's demise with Hepatitis C. Alcohol abuse is widespread in this country, and it's certainly going to be more common among people who've already proven that their coping skills didn't mature along with everybody else's.

The National Institutes of Health state that approximately 10 percent of adults "meet diagnostic criteria for alcohol abuse and alcoholism." I don't think doubling that for Hepatitis C patients is out of order. And, right there we are approaching the 20 to 30 percent of Hepatitis C patients who go on to have life-threatening effects of the disease. Food for thought, no?

People have said to me, "I can't cope with life without drinking alcohol. Can I at least smoke marijuana?" I always say, "Well, it seems like it may be the lesser of two evils, though it has been shown to potentially increase the odds of developing liver cancer even in otherwise healthy people." I'm certainly not advocating the use of controlled substances, but if you've got to do something, marijuana is probably a better choice than alcohol. For Hepatitis C patients, drinking alcohol is like pouring gasoline on a fire.

Alcohol accelerates the progress of liver damage and fibrosis. One study showed cirrhosis to be six times higher in alcoholics with Hepatitis C. Liver cancer rates are also much higher for these people.

Several years ago, I read something that REALLY woke me up to the dangers of alcohol. A new therapy for liver cancer involved isolating a small cluster of cancer cells and injecting a substance directly into those cells that wiped them out immediately. That highly toxic and deadly substance was alcohol. In other words, alcohol is incredibly effective at killing liver cells – rogue cells or otherwise. Yet, even people who should know better drink it all the time.

If, as a Hepatitis C patient, if you can't stop drinking completely when you know it can be life-threatening, then you have a drinking problem and you should seek help. There are plenty of programs (12-step and otherwise) for you to choose from. Plus, there is counseling available from mental health professionals. This is very important. It could save your life.

Let me be perfectly clear. As far as it is known, there is no level of safe alcohol consumption for a Hepatitis C patient. If you find you cannot do without even an occasional drink, then you need some form of assistance and intervention (and there are a variety of potentially helpful programs out there). I highly recommend that you speak with your healthcare provider about this issue. In fact, because it's so harmful to the liver, alcohol use can make you ineligible for medical treatment of Hepatitis C. This may mean that even if you wanted to try the current medical therapy you could not – not as long as you continue to drink alcohol.

The only point of "social drinking" is to get high – to loosen up, relax. Otherwise, holding a glass of seltzer in your hand would do, wouldn't it? There are other, less toxic ways to accomplish this objective, and many don't involve the use of mind or mood altering substances.

If you want to use mood altering substances that are less potentially harmful and more natural than drugs or alcohol, there are herbs and supplements to help you relax and/or sleep. Valerian and skullcap should be avoided if you have liver concerns (even though they are in most natural sleep or relaxation formulas). Find a formula at your health food store that does not contain valerian or skullcap and see if it works for you.

In addition, melatonin and gamma-aminobutyric acid (GABA) are two substances you could ask your local health food store proprietor about. Both work on brain chemicals that help you relax and sleep. They may be of help, depending on how your tension and stress are manifesting. It is not recommended they be used regularly, however, or for long periods of time.

I suggest you check out *The Encyclopedia of Natural Medicine* by Michael Murray, ND and Joseph Pizzorno, ND for even more ideas.

SURVIVAL SECRET

Cigarette smoking can have a direct negative effect on your sick liver.

Regarding tobacco, clinical tests have recently shown that cigarette smoking can exacerbate the liver-harming effects of Hepatitis C. Just consider all the toxins in cigarette smoke, the way nicotine constricts blood vessels and the fact that cigarette smoke has been proven to be a powerful cancer-causing agent. Plus, it seems many people who smoke cigarettes also continue to drink alcohol. So, if you are smoking, please find a way to quit. There are a myriad of programs and methods out there. When it comes to those of us with Hepatitis C quitting cigarette smoking really could be a matter of saving your life – even more so than for the non-infected smoker.

OTHER MUSTS TO AVOID:

Some prescription drugs and over-the-counter medicines should be avoided (if possible) because of their potentially toxic effects on the liver.

Acetaminophen (Tylenol) can be toxic when taken in higher than recommended dosages. Learn more at *http://www.HepCSurvival. com/acetaminophen*. Be sure your doctor takes your Hepatitis C into consideration when recommending or prescribing medications – over-the-counter or otherwise. And, before you try something over-the-counter, ask your doctor about its possible effects on your liver.

All inhaled chemicals can stress the liver. Some that should be avoided completely, or as much as possible, include:

- Chlorine
- Dry cleaning fluids
- Exhaust fumes
- Pesticides
- Paints
- Gasoline and diesel fuel

- Solvents
- Carbon monoxide

It's most important that you protect yourself from these chemicals, especially if you work or live in an environment where you would be exposed to them on a regular basis.

SOCIAL RESPONSE

Survivor Story:

"[The doctor] called me at work and said we needed to talk because I had Hep C. Not knowing the full impact, I started crying, and my boss asked me what was wrong, so I told her. Boy, that was a big mistake. The next day, I came in and there were latex gloves, Lysol, and everybody was sanitizing desks, computers, phones, etc. I was told not to use anybody else's desk."
     – Ellen

Believe it or not, Ellen's story is fairly rare. In my experience, very few people stigmatize Hepatitis C survivors. I heard one story about a husband forbidding his wife from having any contact with her best friend after learning that the friend had Hepatitis C. The irony here is that his wife already had been "exposed" to this person for years after the friend had acquired the disease (but before the diagnosis).

Survivor Story:

"My family doesn't know I have this disease as it would drive my mother crazy everyday and that would, in turn, make me anxious."
     – Chris

I believe there's less stigma, but plenty of confusion, about Hepatitis C. People don't necessarily demonize the illness. They simply don't understand what it's about. If there is a stigma, it has more to do with being "diseased" rather than the particular disease involved. Many people just don't know how to react when they discover you have a chronic and potentially deadly disease. But in general, it doesn't cause family, friends and coworkers to run away and ostracize the patient. More often, it's likely to earn you a hug and a sympathetic ear. However, the odds are at least one person will react negatively. Out of all the people you know, this should hardly matter to you. If you have a problem with this at work, report it to your state employment board.

Survivor Story:

"I am not secretive about having the disease because of concerns about what people might think or how it might affect people or social relationships, because I think getting the word out and stopping the spread of HCV is more important. Yes, I've lost a few friends, but they were not really my friends, they were just acquaintances. If they had been true friends they would have stuck with me, right?"
     – Von

Of course, I have to admit that my status as a Hepatitis C survivor is not something that comes up as the initial topic of conversation. "Hi. Nice to meet you. How about those Yankees? I have Hepatitis C." No, I don't bring it up as the first topic of discussion. In fact, most people don't learn about my condition unless they really get to know me, and then they often don't know what to make of it. So, I usually get to set the tone of the future conversations. "Yeah, I've got a potentially deadly disease, but apparently it's not hurting me too badly. I'm one of the lucky ones. Here are some of the things I'm doing about it..."

Survivor Story:

"I tell everyone who asks. I don't care who knows. Their reaction is their business, not mine. I get lots of exercise, drink lots of water, take milk thistle and live my life."
     – Rob

SURVIVAL SECRET

This one is for your friends and loved ones. Don't share toothbrushes, razors, nail clippers or any other potential source of blood-to-blood contamination.

Carefully follow the advice above, otherwise you could be putting innocent people at risk unnecessarily.

As mentioned earlier, one key area of misunderstanding involves sexual transmission. "Can I transmit it sexually? My partner wants to know." Based on my reading, the chances of contracting the illness through sexual contact are slim to none. However, it's theoretically possible to transfer the disease through sex if there's a blood-to-blood exchange. It depends on what kinds of high-risk behaviors you engage (or have engaged) in. You'll find more info regarding this subject earlier in this book.

I suspect that many people who actually got Hepatitis C by experimenting with intravenous drugs now claim they contracted it through sex. More than 20 years after AIDS first began making headlines, it's more socially acceptable to say that. Well, it's more socially acceptable than admitting you shared a needle with a couple of friends in 1974, anyway.

Survivor Story:

"The only friends/family I have told about this already knew about my high-risk past and I have not told anyone I work with. I feel really sorry for people who got this through transfusions or some other way because I think the general attitude is, 'so what, you are a drug addict and you got what you deserve.'"

– Patricia

Beyond any underlying stigma attached to Hepatitis C, one of the bigger issues – especially among people on PegInterferon-Ribavirin treatments – involves the workplace. If I wanted, I could stuff this book with page after page of case histories I have collected in which people were forced to drastically cut back on hours worked, or had to quit their jobs because of Hepatitis C symptoms or the side effects of combination therapy. In addition, some ignorant bosses will worry that if someone's sick, it's going to cost them money on health insurance, so they may give the patient a hard time in an effort to make them quit.

I know health insurance is often a concern for people with Hepatitis C, if only because it may be difficult to get a new policy when you have a pre-existing condition. In addition, many insurers will not pay for the complementary and alternative therapies discussed earlier in this book. The other issues of concern are how people get treatment if they don't have health insurance and whether the disease entitles you to payments from Medicare or Medicaid. Honestly, I have no professional background with regard to workplace and insurance issues, as well as who is (or is not) entitled to certain government benefits. I've only touched on these topics to make you aware of what you may need to confront. Please research these issues if they apply to you.

SURVIVAL SECRET
Lifestyle changes can count big.

The most important aspect of dealing with this disease is lifestyle modification. Most people need to modify their lifestyle even just to fit the taking of supplements into their schedule on a habitual basis. Even though it could make a huge positive difference, you wouldn't believe the number of people who can't seem to take three capsules of MegaThistle per day, just because they are unaccustomed to making this a part of their lives.

As already stated, regular exercise (at least three or four days per week) is invaluable. Even if you are somewhat debilitated, do what you can to keep your body moving. A little is much better than none. But regularity is keenly important (as with most things of value in life, consistency is more important than intensity). I lift weights, ride my bike, walk and do yoga. In winter I use a "spinning" (stationary) bike. Although I was a runner for 14 years, it just doesn't fit into my lifestyle anymore.

Survivor Story:

"...Abstain from alcohol, exercise daily, drink plenty of water (good water), get a good night's sleep, focus on your spiritual, physical and emotional well-being. I am a pastor, and I have seen many healings in my lifetime. I know that prayer changes things. I know what seems like a crucifixion today can be turned around to be something good at any time. So we do what we can, and the rest is up to God."
     – Peter

Meditation, contemplation and prayer make a real difference in stress management and personal coping mechanism development. Meditation and exercise both help to reduce stress... and as stress seems unavoidable to most of us here in the 21st century, so we need ways to relieve it.

I think it's also important to read inspirational books. Any of the "Chicken Soup" books (or something of that sort) will do. Here are several books that I would highly recommend:

- *Unlimited Power* – Anthony Robbins
- *It's Not What Happens to You It's What You Do About It* – W. Mitchell
- *Healing Words* – Larry Dossey, MD
- *You Can't Afford the Luxury of a Negative Thought* – Peter McWilliams

- *Life 101* – Peter McWilliams and John Roger
- *Radical Healing* – Rudolf Ballentine, MD
- *The Life We Are Given* – George Leonard and Michael Murphy
- *The Little Book of Letting Go* – Hugh Prather
- *Natural Detoxification* – Jacqueline Krohn, MD
- *Timeless Healing, The Power of Biology and Belief* – Herbert Benson, MD
- *Spontaneous Healing* – Andrew Weil, MD
- *Why I Survive AIDS* – Niro Asistent
- *A Brief Explanation of Everything* – Ken Wilbur
- *Doctor's Orders: Go Fishing* – Dean Schrock, Phd.

And don't forget or underestimate the power of laughter. That includes both books of humor and movies/videos. You should be able to acquire any of these by visiting your local library and asking the librarian. Even in my little town, there are county-wide interlibrary loans that put nearly any book or disc I want at my fingertips.

SURVIVAL SECRET
Social support is very important.

DO NOT LET THIS DISEASE ISOLATE YOU

They say a burden shared is a burden halved. Even if your total support network is one friend who is there for you it can make a huge difference in your dealing with this disease.

You can reach out much further, too. In contrast to when I was diagnosed, today there are literally hundreds of support groups around the country. Local and regional groups that have live meetings as well as virtual groups on the internet that provide information, personal interest and emotional support.

You can find support groups online by going to your favorite search engine and typing in "Hepatitis C support group" (you don't need to use the quotation marks and, if you like you can add your city or state to the query. There are also some support groups listed in the resource section of this book. You can also find a support group at *http://www.HepCSurvival.com/support.*

As a fellow Hepatitis C survivor, your health and well-being are important to me. Many people have helped me, and I want to help you. If you have any questions about anything in this chapter, feel free to email me at *Ralph@HepCSurvival.com.*

New information about this disease is becoming available regularly. You can to stay up-to-date by signing up for important email notifications (and a FREE 6-part "survival" e-course) at *http://www.HepCSurvival.com.* This way, I can keep you informed with the latest news, and help you get the most out of this book. You'll also find a multitude of important resources through the website, including my analysis and commentary on new information as I discover it.

CHAPTER 10

Is There Hope for Non-Responders/ Relapsers?

More help is on the way!

I
If you are a non-responder to current medical therapy, perhaps your biggest hope is to use what you've learned earlier in this book to best support and protect yourself and your liver until a better medical treatment is approved. The same is true for any other non-responder you may know. I recently read that 200,000–300,000 people are considered non-responders in the U.S. alone (meaning that they have tried medical treatment and the treatment failed). So at this point what else can you look forward to?

Let's take a look at possible medical treatments on the horizon:

PROTEASE INHIBITORS

One great reason for non-responders to have hope is the ongoing research into additional Hepatitis C-fighting medicines, including protease inhibitors. In a nutshell, these drugs are designed to prevent the Hepatitis C virus from replicating. Current research suggests that Hepatitis C virus (HCV) protease inhibitors could work in tandem with Pegylated Interferon, boosting its effectiveness and possibly allowing for lower doses of Interferon during treatment. Protease inhibitors may also eliminate the need for Ribavirin, which is responsible for the lion's share of side effects. Of course, if you'd prefer a more technical explanation...

"The promise of HCV protease inhibitors (PIs) is in their potential to specifically target HCV, unlike Pegylated Interferon (PegIFN) and Ribavirin (RBV), which work (or fail) through more general antiviral and immune-modulating mechanisms. An effective HCV PI would improve the chances of achieving viral clearance in patients who have not responded to treatment and in groups for whom current therapy is less likely to be successful (including patients with HCV genotype 1, African-Americans, and patients with HIV/HCV co-infection).

"An effective PI might also make treatment more attractive and tolerable by eliminating the need for RBV, shortening the length of treatment, and/or possibly enabling lower doses of PegIFN and, thus, fewer side effects.

"But despite considerable research on HCV PIs over the past decade, it will require at least several more years before an HCV protease inhibitor will win FDA approval and reach the market. Only a few HCV protease inhibitors are currently in human studies, and they are at the very earliest stage of clinical research."[16]

In addition to this particular, albeit indeterminate, hope on the horizon, there are other reasons for optimism. Given the fact that 70 to 80 percent of Hepatitis C patients will not succumb to terrible

16   Raymond, Daniel. "HCV Protease Inhibitors: Glimpses of Hope on a Distant Horizon," International Association of Physicians in AIDS Care, August 2004.

complications, there's a good chance that you may be able to hang in there depending on your condition – even if you do nothing to treat the illness.

Survivor Story:

"Even though therapy didn't work for me, I know that I tried and gave it my best shot. At the present time, my options are limited. I can wait until a new treatment is out that will work for me or I can continue as I am now and hopefully can get on a transplant list. From what I understand you must be in stage 4 before even being considered for transplant. My disease damage has been progressing about a stage per year so, hopefully, by this time next year I will be on the list. For all other survivors, the best advice I can give you is to never give up."
– Susan

AGGRESSIVE HERBAL INTERVENTION?

Aggressive herbal nutritional intervention is yet another cause for hope, especially for people who are slightly symptomatic. As already mentioned, combinations of good multivitamins and minerals, such as vitamins C, E, selenium, N-acetylcysteine (NAC), zinc, some Sho-saiko-to, and good quality phytosome milk thistle (such as MegaThistle) can be a powerful arsenal in protecting and supporting the liver when under attack from the disease. And because most of these approaches have little or no toxicity, you can ramp up the dosages.

At the time of writing, Sho-saiko-to is being studied at the Memorial Sloan Kettering Hospital, specifically for non-responders to Interferon therapies.

In addition, people with more damage to the liver may want to consider adding artichoke, schisandra, licorice root, eclipta alba, pichoriza and other herbs, off and on, as part of a more aggressive nutritional intervention or herbal nutritional intervention.

How do you describe or define "more damage? Well, this is subjective. How do you feel about your condition? How does your doctor feel about your condition? Are you a non-responder? Have you decided not to go with medical therapy, but you're still concerned about your virus? How many things do you want to take in order to counterbalance the symptoms and potential damage until something better comes along? These are questions to ask yourself before testing different regimens.

Do I think everyone should be seeking AGGRESSIVE herbal nutritional intervention? The answer is no – not if your condition is stable and you are otherwise healthy. Personally, I don't need to: A) spend the extra money, and B) spend the extra time taking super-strong supplements three times a day. And, I don't think you need to either. In many cases, lifestyle changes are probably more important than adding a dozen supplements. And, I say this as someone who was instrumental in bringing the phytosome form of milk thistle to the market in an affordable form. This was to best help those with liver concerns. That said, MegaThistle is one supplement I don't EVER plan to stop taking, in addition to the other constituents of my "A-List" (refer to page 126). It is my considered opinion that these supplements are essential to my continued health.

MAKE UP YOUR OWN MIND

As a Hepatitis C survivor, I'm not about pushing more herbal products. I recommend what's worked for me, and provide information to others like me so they can make up their own minds. I will never claim that you NEED a particular herbal product – or any combination thereof. I will never say that you NEED to undertake conventional therapy or avoid it. I just know it's not for me at this time. Be aware of what's working (or not) for other people before reaching your own conclusions.

I've spoken directly with hundreds of Hepatitis C patients whose regimens are similar to mine, as well as hundreds whose treatments are different from mine. You need to learn as much as you can and then determine what you need to do for yourself.

My personal situation is one of the chicken and the egg. The "egg" (or was it the "chicken"?) was that I needed to do something for my Hepatitis C. And then, when I discovered a milk thistle extract that beats every other milk thistle extract hands-down, I made it available to others at a much more reasonable price than it was before. And now I'm doing the same again with MegaThistle. All of my subsequent research has come about as a result of my involvement with that particular product, which has led me to search for other products and treatments that may help Hepatitis C survivors lead healthier, more productive lives; which I've clearly outlined here in this book.

If you choose to forgo herbal intervention, that's okay with me. If you choose a product or treatment based on the information provided in this book, that's okay too. If you choose (say) a milk thistle product, and don't buy the best quality and formulation at the cheapest price, I don't mind – I really don't. Although I know you would do better with MegaThistle.

As seminar facilitators often say, "If you're going to take away one point from today's discussion, let it be this: DON'T DO ANYTHING RASH!" Please, do not do anything rash based on your diagnosis. To start, get more information to determine your prognosis. Learn your genotype, your viral load, your AST, your ALT and other enzyme levels.

You might ask, don't people normally receive this information when they're diagnosed? Not necessarily. Some people still don't learn their viral load or genotype. And that's really crazy. Some physicians may not volunteer this information, because they believe there's only one approved conventional treatment, so they think, "What difference does it make to determine genotype and viral loads? If the person has Hepatitis C, I can only treat with combination therapy, so what's the difference? I'll check that other stuff just before we begin treatment so we'll have some baselines."

Be cautious and do not blindly follow your doctor's recommendations. Also, do not follow the advice of herbal purveyors blindly. You must take some responsibility to weigh and measure what's sensible, what's affordable, and what's most likely to help your condition.

Survivor Story:

"*I count myself lucky on many fronts. I have a supportive family, friends, work, and insurance situation. I had a treatment-responsive genotype of the virus (2b), and I caught it before cirrhosis had set in. But the best thing that happened was I learned how to slow down and appreciate my family and good friends. I cut out the relationships that were superficial, and concentrated on the ones that meant the most to me. Before, I was constantly on the go, with lots of commitments. It wasn't easy, especially at first, when people who had always known me as healthy and sociable were reluctant to let go. My friends at work, for instance, didn't understand that while I may have wanted to go to lunch with them, eating in and resting during my lunch hour served me better.*"

– Sharon

Take responsibility for your health. Do what you can to support and protect your liver and immune system. Only after that should you start looking at treatments that may be more radical (conventional or otherwise). If you do things that are bad for your liver, you first need to stop doing them, and then start doing something good for your liver. Most people know what to do, but they just don't bother to make the necessary lifestyle changes. This involves willpower and consciousness – thinking differently, eating differently, drinking differently, and dealing with stress differently. It's all about living differently. Unfortunately, most people are slaves to inertia, and do what they've always done. That's one reason Thoreau said, "Most men lead lives of quiet desperation."

You need to be brave to change. You need to want to live differently. You need to want to live. Most people are stuck with just getting by. There is nothing wrong with asking for help. There are professionals who can assist in lifestyle and behavior modification. Don't be shy. If you need help, seek it out.

MORE PROMISING THERAPIES ON THE HORIZON
New Interferons:

Targeted anti-viral drugs, anti-fibrotics, new forms of Interferon and other therapies are being studied, and some look very promising.

Albuferon (albInterferon alpha-2b) is one that is being studied because it seems to be as effective as Pegylated Interferon but may only need to be given half as often to achieve comparable results.

Ribavirin substitutes: These are being investigated because of the potentially severe side effects of Ribavirin as it exists today.

Viramidine (also known as taribalirin) is a substance which is turned into Ribavirin in the liver and is therefore found to have fewer side effects. Testing so far has shown it may be as effective against HCV as standard oral Ribavirin.

Protease inhibitors: All are currently being developed against genotype 1, the hardest to fight with current means.
BILN 2061 showed great promise against the virus but was also found to be potentially cardiotoxic (poisonous to the heart tissues). For this reason research has stalled on this one.

VX-950 (Teleprevir) has shown to be marginally effective as a monotherapy. In one test with Interferon and Ribavirin against genotype 1 it showed that 12 out of 12 patients got a sustained viral response after just 28 days of treatment. As of March 2009 it was announced that VX-950 was four times as effective in half the time in "curing" previous genotype 1 non-responders. This is huge! More studies are being conducted (and the results anxiously awaited by HCV patients everywhere).

ITMN 191 (the protease inhibitor) being developed by InterMune has been shown to be active against proteases from genotypes 1, 2 and 3. It is orally administered, and according to a November 2008 press release, it will be tested further with another oral agent, R7128, which is a polymerase inhibitor.

In January 2009, Pharmasset Inc. and Roche Pharmaceuticals announced a phase 2b trial of R7128 to complement the study of R7227 (ITMN-191) and R7128 at the same time. Indix Pharmaceuticals initiated a study of IDX184 – a liver-targeted nucleotide pro-drug candidate. It is a once-daily oral treatment.

Polymerase inhibitors: NM-283 (Valopicitabine) received much attention initially. It seemed to have promise but had considerable limitations. In fact, Idenix suspended testing in July 2007 indefinitely. But, as others enter this particular area, it is looking like another one of hope for better therapies in the future. For instance, Pharmasset Inc. and Roche announced ongoing studies of R7-128, a pro-drug of PSI-6130; a cytodine nucleoside analog inhibitor of HCV RNA Polymerase R7227 (ITMN-191), a protease inhibitor.

Viral Protein Antagonists: Many other pharmaceutical companies are working on this area with potential to develop new treatment candidates.

A P O T E N T I A L   G I F T

This disease, like anything else in life, can be a gift. Use it to examine your behaviors, your relationships, your spiritual connection, your sense of community, your compassion, your forgiveness, your love, your death, your values, your dreams, your desires, your fears, your priorities, your accomplishments, your shortcomings, and your hopes. It is a wake up call. You are mortal – life is fragile, and when all is said and done, whether you live 10 more years or 100 more, what really matters to you? Life is not about the years lived, but the moments enjoyed.

Too many of us live our lives based on old patterns, not deliberate actions. If you look at the word "deliberate," it's quite interesting. In its Latin roots, it means "of liberation." Yet we interpret it to mean "to think deeply and carefully about." This is because thinking deeply and carefully about things liberates you to live your life with clarity and integrity.

Deliberation should be part of all your decisions. The word "decision," when literally translated from the Latin, means "to cut off from." When we truly decide to do one thing, we are equally deciding not to do another. A wholesome, fulfilling life is not about fence sitting. It's about making deliberate decisions and taking action.

SURVIVAL SECRET

Hepatitis C patients can still be organ donors.

There are not enough livers or other organs donated to save everyone in need. Even with HCV you can be a donor. Consider this; if something were to happen to you that took your life suddenly, your liver might go on to save the life of another HCV patient. So be sure to sign an organ donor card, and let your relatives know.

LIVER TRANSPLANTATION:
WHEN ALL ELSE FAILS...

According to a computer simulation model, the number of chronic liver disease deaths from HCV will increase from 8,000 to 10,000 per year currently to approximately 19,300 per year between 2010 and 2019.

Liver transplantation is often a final treatment option for long-term progressive liver disease. Nationally, 89 percent of liver transplant patients are alive one year after surgery. The first obstacle to overcome is the long wait for a donor liver. It can be up to two years, so many doctors may begin speaking to you about this option well before it is nearly necessary.

According to the Mayo Clinic, approximately 15,00 to 17,000 people are waiting to receive a liver transplant on any given day. Annually, though, there are only enough livers (donated by those who have passed on) for about a third of them. Recently, in July 2009, much was made of Steve Jobs' liver transplant. Many people feel that ethically, having power, money or position should not put people higher up on the list. The same situation was an issue when Mickey Mantle, the baseball great, got a "go to the head of the liver queue" pass.

Live donor transplants are becoming more common for this very reason, as well as the fact that they are gaining acceptance in the medical community and in the public at large. A person (usually a direct family member) can donate a portion of their liver in a process not unlike donating one kidney. Only, unlike with the kidney, the donor liver grows back the missing portion within weeks of surgery.

For a full liver transplant, the surgery takes three to five hours to perform, and includes a five to ten day hospital stay. The patient is then treated with immune system suppressants so they do not reject the new organ. These drugs can cause their own problems, but, thanks to the transplant you are actually around to deal with these problems.

Clearly, if your doctor begins to speak with you about transplantation it's time to do your homework and learn all you can about specialized transplantation centers in your geographic area, insurance coverage, recommended doctors, and other issues.

Reading the information here may also inspire you to donate your own organs and possibly encourage your friends and relatives to do the same.

The U.S. Department of Health and Human Services sent the following press release addressing this issue:

U.S. Public Is Taking Action to Support Organ Donation, Gallup Survey Finds

HHS's Health Resources and Services Administration (HRSA) today announced the results of a 2005 Gallup Organization survey which indicates that Americans continue to strongly support the donation of organs and tissues for transplantation. More importantly, the survey also finds that far higher percentages of Americans have taken personal actions to become organ donors since a similar 1993 survey on donation.

The percentage of individuals who have granted permission to donate their organs or tissues on a driver's license or an organ donor card reached 53 percent in 2005, almost double the 28 percent who had done so in 1993. HRSA Administrator Elizabeth Duke urges anyone interested in becoming an organ donor to learn how at *http://www. OrganDonor.gov*. HRSA directs federal efforts to promote donation.

Nearly all of the survey respondents – 97 percent – said they would donate a family member's organs if they knew the person's wishes ahead of time. The 2005 survey reported that 71 percent of Americans had talked to a family member about their donation wishes, up from 52 percent in 1993.

"Make sure you tell your relatives about your intention to donate once you sign up. Sharing your intentions with family members is an important part of the donation process," Duke added.

Gallup also found that among U.S. racial and ethnic groups, Whites (61 percent) in 2005 were most likely to indicate donation on their driver's license, followed by Latinos and Asians (both at 39 percent), and Blacks (31 percent).

"The results of this survey show that more Americans than ever are aware of the importance of organ donation and are taking action," stated Duke. "But we must do more, particularly in minority communities where support for donation is weaker. I encourage more families to discuss this issue, because their decision to donate in a time of grief can bring hope and life to many others."

The Gallup Organization's 2005 National Survey of Organ and Tissue Donation Attitudes and Behaviors questioned over 2,000 Americans concerning their attitudes toward donation of organs and tissues for transplantation. The study replicates the 1993 survey and includes new items as well. For more information on how you can become an organ donor and more detail on the Gallup survey results, visit *http://www.organdonor.gov/survey2005*.

In my opinion, the most significant fact in this press release is that 97 percent would donate a relative's organs if they knew that was the wish of the relative. So, it is not enough to fill out a donor card or have it put on your driver's license. Family members and other loved ones also need to be told of your wishes.

IN CONCLUSION

As a fellow Hepatitis C survivor it is my hope you found real value in the pages of this book. For not much more than the cost of an insurance co-pay for a 10-minute visit to the doctor, you got one heck of a lot more information, that's for sure. Just one tip or suggestion that helps you cope or adjust more appropriately to your condition should be worth many times your investment of time and money in reading this book.

As mentioned earlier, if you would like to read the full text survivor stories the excerpts in this book were taken from (hundreds were submitted) you can go to *http://www.HepCSurvival.com/stories* where I will be posting selected ones on an ongoing basis. While you are there you can also add your own story to inform and help others, if you like, or even comment on those submitted by others.

FINAL SURVIVAL SECRET

You can help save lives by suggesting more people you meet get tested for Hepatitis C.

The Centers for Disease Control estimates perhaps half the people with chronic Hepatitis C don't even know they have it. That equates to up to two million people in the United States. Which means they may be putting themselves at greater risk by lifestyle choices they are making. If they find out they have it they can start learning more and making informed decisions about how they want to handle the disease and handle their own survival.

As a fellow Hepatitis C survivor, your health and well-being are important to me. Many people have helped me, and I want to help you. If you have any questions about anything in this chapter, feel free to email me at *Ralph@HepCSurvival.com*. New information about this disease is becoming available regularly. You can to stay up-to-date by signing up for important email notifications (and a FREE 6-part "survival" e-course) at *http://www.HepCSurvival.com*. This way, I can keep you informed with the latest news, and help you get the most out of this book. You'll also find a multitude of important resources through the website, including my analysis and commentary on new information as I discover it.

Resources

The following websites offer a wealth of articles on Hepatitis C approaches, both conventional and alternative, as well as research studies and other information that can help you determine how best to treat your illness. The list is not exhaustive, but features some of the best websites I've encountered. There are also some other books listed you may find useful.

- *www.liverhealthtoday.org* (the only magazine dedicated to Hepatitis C patients and their families)
- *www.hepatitisneighborhood.com* (many resources and support options)
- *www.hepc-connection.org* (a very active and professional non-profit working for the benefit of Hepatitis C patients)
- *www.hivandhepatitis.com* (chock-full of current information and commentary)
- *www.nccam.nih.gov* (website for the NIH's National Center for Complementary and Alternative Medicine)
- *www.nlm.gov/medlineplus/hepatitisc.html* (an online service provided by the National Library of Medicine)
- *www.quackwatch.org* (website of a nonprofit corporation "whose purpose is to combat health-related frauds, myths, fads, fallacies, and misconduct")
- *www.cdc.gov* (website of the Centers for Disease Control and Prevention)
- *www.hcvadvocate.org* (website of the Hepatitis C Support Project)
- *www.nationalhepatitis-c.org* (website of the National Hepatitis C Coalition)
- *www.healthyhepper.com* (with a great support group, HepCWarriors)
- *www.hepcchallenge.org* (The website of the Hepatitis C Caring Ambassadors Program. Very helpful.)
- *www.hcvets.com* (excellent info on Hepatitis C among U.S. Military Veterans)
- Additional books you may find useful:
    Living With Hepatitis C For Dummies by Nina L. Paul, Gina Pollichino
    Hepatitis C Cookbook: Easy and Delicious Recipes by Heather Jeanne
    The Hepatitis C Handbook by Matthew Dolan, Iain Murray-Lyon, and John Tindall
    Dr. Melissa Palmer's Guide To Hepatitis and Liver Disease by Melissa Palmer
    The Hepatitis C Help Book, by Misha Ruth Cohen O.M.D. L. Ac., Robert Gish, and Kalia Doner
    Living with Hepatitis C: A Survivor's Guide by Gregory T. Everson

ABOUT THE AUTHOR

Ralph Napolitano has been a licensed healthcare provider in New York State for more than 25 years, though his study of holistic and complementary medicine predates that by many years. He is also a Hepatitis C survivor.

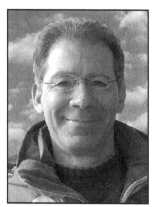

Ralph Napolitano

As an avid runner for 14 years, Ralph learned a great deal about how to enhance his health and improve his running. He did most of this through nutrition, yoga, and cross-training, including swimming, biking, calisthenics and free-weights.

Ralph worked in a health-food store back in 1975 (when they were still quite rare). It was there he began to learn about natural foods and supplements. Ralph also became a fitness trainer at one of the foremost health clubs in the country. Studying to become a licensed healthcare provider in New York State during the early 1980's gave him a deep grounding in anatomy and physiology (and even cellular biology and biochemistry).

Also during the 1980's Ralph hosted a popular cable television program where he interviewed numerous recognized experts in the natural health field, such as Dr. Frank Lipman, Dr. Leo Galland, Dr. Peter D'Adamo, Dr. Jefferey Moss, Dr. Linda Rector-Page and many others.

In 1996 he co-founded a leading healthcare institute and authored/ published courses for healthcare professionals which have been studied by thousands worldwide.

In 1999 he started a website to help other Hepatitis C patients gain affordable access to the most powerful and helpful milk thistle formulas on the market.

In 2002, Ralph took the helm of a major hepatitis authority website after its founder decided to pursue other interests. He did this in order to ensure that thousands of pages of valuable online information remained available for patients.

As the main point of contact at the websites, Ralph has communicated with thousands of Hepatitis C patients. Through this avenue he learned what the prevailing questions and concerns of survivors were. Comments from some of these patients appear in this book, with permission.

He has since left the company he co-founded. He has gone back partially to his private practice as a licensed healthcare professional in New York State, and is rededicating himself to helping those with Hepatitis C.

By communicating with so many patients while at his earlier company and focusing on Hepatitis C for nearly twenty years, Ralph has acquired a sense of the type of information still sorely needed by the Hepatitis C community. This book is a contribution to fulfilling that need. Reading this book is just the beginning for you, though. Much of what is covered in these pages is supplemented by much more in-depth information on the companion website, *http://www.HepCSurvival.com.*

Also, there is new information frequently becoming available regarding health, nutrition, Hepatitis C, medical treatments, etc. Ralph makes a point of keeping up with this updated information, and wants to help you do the same. Just go to the website, *http://www.HepCSurvival. com* and sign up for regular email updates. Not only will you be given the most recent information, but Ralph will also provide commentary and clarification to help put it all into perspective for you. This way, you will be able to make better choices regarding your own personal situation.

One last thing: as part of his dedication to others who share his affliction, Ralph invites you to contact him either through email or on the website. Please don't hesitate to do so. He simply requests that you have read this book from cover-to-cover so he needn't spend unnecessary time on information he has already shared here.

As a fellow Hepatitis C survivor, your health and well-being are important to me. Many people have helped me, and I want to help you. If you have any questions about anything in this chapter, feel free to email me at *Ralph@HepCSurvival.com.*
New information about this disease is becoming available regularly. You can to stay up-to-date by signing up for important email notifications (and a FREE 6-part "survival" e-course) at *http://www.HepCSurvival.com.* This way, I can keep you informed with the latest news, and help you get the most out of this book. You'll also find a multitude of important resources through the website, including my analysis and commentary on new information as I discover it.

INDEX

conventional/medical approach in, 10, 11
do-nothing approach, 11, 41-42
guidelines for, 86-87
health insurance issues in, 160
non-responders to (See Non-responders)
questions to ask, 168
responsibility for, 169, 170
therapies on the horizon, 171-172
time to initiation of, 18
of whole person, 65
Triglyceride levels, high fructose corn syrup and, 108
Tumeric extract, for inflammation, 128

U
Ultrasound, for fibrosis evaluation, 26, 27
UV treatment, 92-94

V
Vaccination, importance of, 14
Valerian, avoidance of, 155
Valopictabine (NM-283), 172
Vata, 72
Vegetables
  cooked, 111
  cruciferous, 112
  fresh vs. canned, 110-111
  raw vs. cooked, 111
Viral load
  expression of, 25
  in genotype 1 patients, 29
  HCV ribonucleic acid test for, 24-25
  relation to liver damage, 29-30
  treatment options and, 28
Viramidine, 171
Viruses, reproduction methods of, 13
Vitamin A
  as antioxidant, 123
  maximum dosage of, 142

Vitamin C
  as antioxidant, 123, 124, 130
  buffered form of, 130
  dosage of, 130
Vitamin D-3, 133-134
  deficiency of, 134
  maximum dosage of, 142
Vitamin E
  as antioxidant, 123, 124
  dosage of, 130
Vitamins, 123
  antioxidant, 123, 124, 130
  multi-vitamin preparation, 130
VX-950 (Teleprivir), 171

W
Walking, 147-148
  optimum minimum of, 148
Water
  daily intake of, 113, 117
  pegInterferon-Ribavirin therapy and, 113, 117
Workplace, stigma in, 157

X
Xiao-chai-hu-tang
  compared to Sho-saiko-to, 69, 70
  milk thistle cost comparison with, 71

Y
Yoga, 149, 150

Z
"Zappers," Hulda Clark's, 92
Zinc
  as antioxidant, 123, 124
  as antiviral, 133
  dosage of, 133

Dear Reader,

Discover a powerful way for you to get even more value out of **Hepatitis C Survival Secrets:**

With you in mind, I've developed a no-cost e-course entitled, **"The Six Essential Hep C Survival Shortcuts."**

You see, at this point I'm assuming you've fully read this book and gotten lots of ideas from it. Now, the question becomes, what do you do next? And after that, then what?

To help you to implement positive health-enhancing changes much more easily and systematically into your life, I've compiled the most useful suggestions from the book into a six part, step-by-step program.

In order to claim this valuable gift for yourself, go to **http://www.hepcsurvival.com** where you will find instructions for accessing this highly useful bonus.

Site visitors who haven't read the book will be advised to do so to get maximum benefit from this e-course.

The course is intended to help you get the most out of the important ideas covered in this book. The value of this bonus alone is $97, but you get it at no charge.

This course is my special gift to you, my fellow Hepatitis C survivor, for investing in yourself, in this book, and in me.

Be well,

Ralph Napolitano

Made in the USA
Lexington, KY
27 April 2013